STRENGTH
TRAINING
for
SENIORS

T0116683

STRENGTH TRAINING
for
SENIORS

INCREASE YOUR BALANCE,
STABILITY, AND STAMINA TO REWIND
THE AGING PROCESS

PAIGE WAEHNER

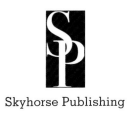

Skyhorse Publishing

Skyhorse Publishing books may be purchased in bulk at special discounts for sales promotion, corporate gifts, fund-raising, or educational purposes. Special editions can also be created to specifications. For details, contact the Special Sales Department, Skyhorse Publishing, 307 West 36th Street, 11th Floor, New York, NY 10018 or info@skyhorsepublishing.com.

Skyhorse® and Skyhorse Publishing® are registered trademarks of Skyhorse Publishing, Inc.®, a Delaware corporation.

Visit our website at www.skyhorsepublishing.com.

10 9 8 7 6

Library of Congress Cataloging-in-Publication Data is available on file.

Cover design by Mona Lin
Cover photo credit: Getty Images

ISBN: 978-1-5107-5895-7
Ebook ISBN: 978-1-5107-5897-1

Printed in China

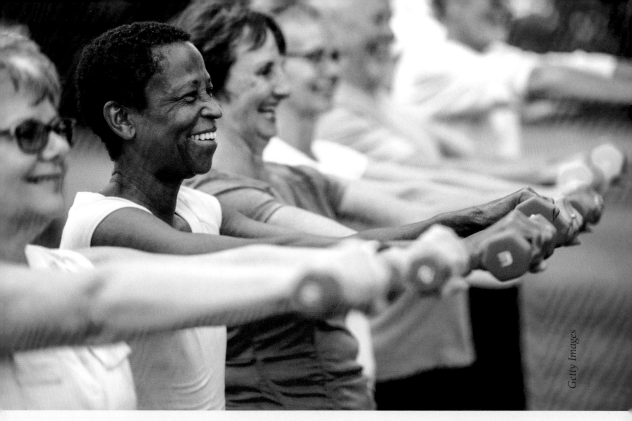

Getty Images

Contents

Introduction: The Importance of Strength Training for Older Adults

What would you do to gain access to the Fountain of Youth? People have been searching for this mythical artifact for centuries. There have been stories of healing rivers going back to the fourth century BCE, the most notable being the legend that the Spanish explorer Ponce de León was actually searching for the Fountain of Youth when he landed in Florida in 1513.

Historians now assert that this was not the real reason for his travels, but through the years many people have believed in the restorative power of "magical" waters.

These days, we know the real Fountain of Youth doesn't exist (at least we think so), but that doesn't mean there isn't a way to increase longevity as well as the quality of life as we age.

In fact, there is a way to reverse the aging process all the way down to the cellular level: strength training.

We can't stop the aging process, which is determined by our genes, but there are other factors that affect how we age such as nutrition, stress, smoking, and exercise.

By focusing on these things, especially strength training, your biological age may just end up being a lot younger than your chronological age. That means not just living longer, but enjoying living longer.

Whether you're already active and exercising or it's been a while, this book will show you exactly what you need to do to work on building lean muscle tissue, strength, and stamina. You'll also work on some of the most important aspects that your body needs to age well and avoid injuries and falls: balance, core strength, and stability.

And the best part is that it's never too late to start! While defining what a "senior" population is can be a complex process, experts generally start with the youngest baby boomers, born in 1964, and includes anyone up to more than 100 years old.

But, no matter how old you are or what your fitness level is now, anyone can get stronger. Studies show that for seniors, starting weight training helps you avoid age-related muscle loss, which is integral for being strong, being independent, and preventing injuries.

Your life will get easier. Chasing after kids or grandkids, carrying groceries, getting in and out of a car, cleaning, and chores will all get easier when you're strong, and it's not just about physical strength. Strength training builds confidence and helps combat mental health concerns like anxiety and depression.

My own interest in working with seniors began with my grandmother. In her 80s, she was still doing water aerobics and riding a stationary bike at the local YMCA. At some point, she stopped going and, within a year, she could barely walk with a walker. She fell and broke her hip and, within the next few months, at 89, she passed away.

She lived a great life, of course, but it really brought home to me just how much a little strength can go such a long way. With regular exercise, she might have been healthier, happier, and more independent. Her decline may not have been so fast, and maybe I would have had her in my life a little longer.

Weight training has helped me through so many things, from regular life events like having to bail water out of my basement during a flood to healing from four different back surgeries. It has helped me in so many ways, and I want that for you, too. This is the prime of your life, so let's make it as good as we can!

By opening this book, you've started on your path to a new, stronger body. I promise to walk you through a scientifically-backed 12-week program that helps you gradually and safely build strength, muscle, balance, stability, and more. I can't wait to get started.

Chapter 1
The Basics of Resistance Training

Resistance training has been around for about as long as civilization. In fact, go back to ancient Rome and Greece and you find the origins of the Olympics which highlighted strength, power, and speed with such sports as the discus, shot put, or the hammer throw.

Throughout time, resistance training has evolved to fit our modern world with equipment such as dumbbells, barbells, weight machines, and more.

Our understanding of resistance training has evolved as well. While it was once considered for bodybuilders like Arnold Schwarzenegger, we now know that anyone can benefit from lifting weights, especially older adults.

What experts have figured out through a variety of studies is that if we lift enough weight for a certain number of repetitions and sets of an exercise, we can build muscle and strength.

And it's not just muscles that benefit. We also know that resistance training can help build stronger bones, a great benefit for anyone but especially people dealing with osteoporosis.

So why is all of this so important?

Think of an everyday activity, such as moving from a seated to a standing position, something many of us do throughout the day. That one activity involves a variety of muscles:

The quadriceps, on the front of the thighs and the glutes, shorten and contract to help your body stand against gravity. And, those aren't the only muscles working. Your core muscles work to keep you balanced and then there are your feet, ankles, and calves also working at the same time.

Think of how many times you do that in one day, sitting and standing, and all the important muscles used for that simple activity.

Making those muscles stronger makes that activity easier, just one reason that resistance training can actually improve your daily life. It's not just resistance training, but functional training.

That said, resistance training has some basic tenets to help you understand how it works and how to create workouts that make sense for your needs and goals.

a. The Exercises—The first thing to understand about resistance training is that we want to focus on all the major muscle groups in the body. In fact, during the first few weeks of this program, that's exactly what you're going to work on. Those include:

    i. Chest—These are some of the largest muscles in the upper body used for pushing motions such as pushing open a door. Just a few exercises you'll do to work the chest include push-ups, chest presses, and chest flies.

    ii. Back—The back also includes large, strong muscles, especially the latissimus dorsi (the lats) on either side of the back. You use these muscles to pull things towards you and the exercises mimic that, such as dumbbell rows and reverse flies. We'll also focus on the lower back, which is one area of the body that often feels stiff and sore from a little too much sitting.

    iii. Shoulders—The shoulders are involved in everything from lifting things overhead to pulling on a seatbelt. The exercises that target these muscles include overhead presses, lateral raises, and upright rows.

    iv. Biceps—Think of picking up a set of grocery bags and holding them as you walk to your door. Your biceps are doing most of the work here and you'll do a variety of exercises, from biceps curls to concentration curls, to build endurance and strength in your arms.

    v. Triceps—The back of your arms include three small muscles called the triceps and these are involved in any pushing motion. You'll do kickbacks and triceps extensions to work these muscles, making them stronger in daily life.

    vi. Core—Many people think the core only involves the abdominal muscles, but it actually includes your entire torso, including your abs, lower back, and pelvic area. Consider your core as your powerhouse, the origin of all basic movements and, of course, the muscles that protect your spine. You'll do a variety of specific exercises to keep your core lean and strong for all your daily movements.

vii. Lower body—Your hips, glutes, thighs, calves, and feet are the bedrock of your body and where much of your strength comes from, whether you're walking to the mailbox or getting in and out of your car. The lower body exercises you'll do in this program, along with balance training, will give you such a strong base; there's nothing you won't be able to do.

b. Types of Resistance—The next part of resistance training is, of course, using something that challenges your muscles so that they can respond by growing stronger. That resistance can be your body weight, which will be something we focus on in the first few weeks of training. Beyond that, it can open up to include almost anything that adds weight to your exercises. This can include:

i. Dumbbells—Hand weights are the very foundation of basic strength training. They're versatile, inexpensive, and you can use them for a variety of exercises. In this program, you'll learn what weights you need and how to use them for different exercises.

ii. Barbells—While these aren't included in this program, barbells may be something you choose to use in the future to up your game. These are adjustable weights that allow you to lift heavier and adapt to different exercises depending on your strength and fitness level. They usually come with a bar and a set of weighted plates that you can exchange depending on the exercise you're doing.

iii. Resistance bands—These flexible bands are excellent for building both strength and endurance. They're a favorite of mine because they're inexpensive, take up very little room, and can be used for almost any exercise. What I like is that bands create a kind of tension you don't experience with other types of equipment, firing your muscle fibers in a whole new way. You'll use these throughout the program to add a more dynamic feel to some of your exercises.

iv. Medicine balls—These aren't part of this particular program, but weighted balls can be used in place of almost any weighted exercise, giving you a different way to work your muscles.

v. Machines—Machines, whether you use them at home or at the gym, are also a great choice for adding resistance to different exercises. These are often a great fit for beginners because the machines are designed to guide you through the proper movement and you can typically use heavier weights because machines provide added support for your body.

c. Repetitions and Sets—Once you get your exercises and resistance sorted out, there's the question of how many repetitions (reps) you do of an exercise as well as how many sets. The reps refer to how many times you do an exercise (say a biceps curl), while a set refers to how many times you do that exercise (say, one set of ten biceps curls). The idea behind this is that there is a range of repetitions of an exercise that will give you the most bang for your buck. And beyond that, you're looking at diminishing returns.

   i. Repetition ranges: What experts have found is that there's a range of repetitions that serve different goals. These typically apply to athletes who want to compete in bodybuilding competitions or athletes excelling at other sports. Over time and with further studies, experts have found the different rep ranges to apply to almost any goal:

      » 6-12 reps: This goes into the bodybuilder category where your goal is to build larger muscles as well as build strength. With those goals, you lift as much as you can for those reps, meaning the very last rep is usually the very last rep one can do with good form.

      » 8-12 reps: Here we get into the middle ground of weight training, with a focus on building muscle and strength and, for those of us without a competition in the works, this is the sweet spot of strength training.

      » 12-16 reps: For this rep range, the focus is on building endurance, although you can also build strength and muscle within this range. This range is ideal for those of us working on balance, stability, strength, and endurance and you'll find that many of the exercises you do within this program fall within this range.

ii. Sets: Just as experts have studied just how many repetitions you do per exercise, they also know that doing a certain number of sets can make a difference in strength and fitness. For older adults, as well as any new exerciser, experts agree that starting out with one set is usually enough stimulus to build strength and muscle. You'll find that, throughout the program, you'll start each workout with one set and progress to two sets in the following time period.

d. Rest Between Sets—One other aspect of strength training involves resting between sets. This is a question many new exercisers have: If you're going to do 10 reps of an exercise, then rest and do another 10 reps, why not do 20 reps? It's a good question and one that experts have figured out. The point of resting between sets is to maximize your muscle's time under tension for those reps. Once those muscles are fatigued, you give them a break to recover and then do the next set, which is how you build more strength and endurance. For heavy lifters, the rest between sets can be several minutes but for those of us wanting to get fit and strong, that rest period is usually much shorter, between 10 and 60 seconds.

e. Recovery Days—While working out is important, what's even more important is taking time to rest and recover between workouts. This is especially true of strength training workouts because here's one thing to understand: You don't want to work the same muscles two days in a row. That means, if you work your arms today, you want to give yourself at least a day before you work them again. That time allows your muscles to recover and grow. This knowledge helps us create a workout schedule that allows for maximum growth while also building in rest periods.

Chapter 2

Why You Should Lift Weights

There are so many reasons you should lift weights—that could be a whole separate book. For a lot of us growing up, it was either something we did in gym class because we had to or something competitors did. The average person didn't even consider lifting weights for any reason.

Now we know that, at its basic level, lifting weights resonates within our very cells. There are structural changes that happen at the cellular level that lead to some of our biggest challenges as we grow older. It often feels inevitable but, believe it or not, there are things we can do about some of these changes and, yes, it starts in the cells of our bodies.

There are functional consequences of aging that most of us have probably experienced once we get past forty. These consequences include reductions in:

- ✓ Accuracy
- ✓ Speed
- ✓ Range
- ✓ Endurance
- ✓ Coordination
- ✓ Stability
- ✓ Strength
- ✓ Flexibility

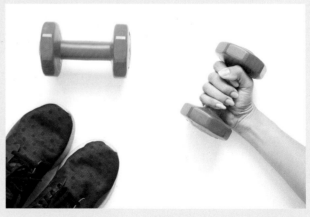

All of these physical facets affect our daily lives and determine just how independent we are as we get older. In fact, low activity levels end up causing physical declines that, eventually, can lead to frailty.

Getty Images

Frailty is a state of vulnerability which is caused by functional impairment of everyday activities. This is also associated with sarcopenia, which is the loss of muscle mass that can happen with age.

Now on to the good news: your personal Fountain of Youth—resistance training—creates all kinds of great things that happen both inside your body and out, right away and over time.

IMMEDIATE BENEFITS:

- ✓ **Stable blood sugar levels**—Exercise actually helps your body regulate blood sugar levels. This is good for a variety of reasons, but the most important one is that you have a constant source of energy running through your body rather than having spikes that could affect your ability to function.
- ✓ **Increase in "feel-good" hormones**—These hormones, like adrenaline and noradrenaline, are stimulated by exercise and give you instant energy and often a boost in your mood.
- ✓ **Improved sleep**—Studies have shown that regular exercise can help your quality of sleep at all ages, especially if you workout in the morning.
- ✓ **Increase your metabolism**—An increased metabolism is great for losing weight, if that's a goal you are working toward, which means you're burning more calories just doing daily activities.
- ✓ **Lowers blood pressure**—It's normal for many of us to be diagnosed with high blood pressure as we get older and exercise is one thing that can help manage this, both in the short-term and the long-term.
- ✓ **Decreased arthritis pain**—It may seem counterintuitive to exercise if you're in pain, but when you strengthen the muscles around the joints with arthritis, you may feel an improvement within just two weeks of starting your exercise program. In addition, when you exercise, you warm the blood going to the muscles and joints, which also helps reduce pain and stiffness.

THE LONG-TERM BENEFITS

Exercising over time can improve almost every function in your body, and it doesn't take much exercise to make a difference. One of the most important benefits from exercise is more about protection rather than some of the more visible goals like weight loss.

In fact, many of the benefits we get from exercise are things that are hard to see or measure, which is just one reason it's sometimes hard to find the motivation to work out, even when we know it's good for us.

CARDIOVASCULAR FUNCTION

For people who don't exercise regularly, cardiovascular function can decline as they get older. This involves how much blood your heart pumps to the body as well as how much oxygen can make it to your muscles. Exercising can increase your heart's efficiency, which means you can do more, protect your heart, and feel good all at the same time.

LUNG STRENGTH AND CAPACITY

The efficiency of your breathing can decline with age, and some of this is due to the degeneration of the discs in the spine, which affects the muscles surrounding your lungs. This means that you have less lung capacity, something you may not even realize. Exercise can help reduce the speed of degeneration in the spine, which means breathing better and easier.

BLOOD PRESSURE

Blood pressure increases with age, with some studies showing that about 75 percent of Americans over the age of 75 have high blood pressure.

Here's the good news: studies show that in middle-aged and older adults, exercise capacity is a very strong predictor of whether you have a small elevation of blood pressure or whether you actually have hypertension, something that could lead to heart disease, strokes, and other problems. The other good news here is that all exercise counts, so even just a few minutes of extra walking a day can make a difference.

MUSCLE STRENGTH AND ENDURANCE

Now here's where the real benefits come in, because while you can't always feel the decline in cardiovascular function or lung capacity, you can definitely feel the benefits of being stronger and fitter.

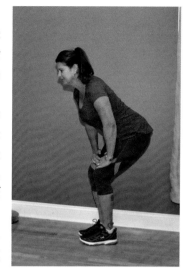

Experts know that strength and endurance decline with age. Loss of muscle function is usually due to the loss of muscle mass. Here's the important part: if you're sedentary, your muscle mass can decline by about 22 to 23 percent for men and women between the ages of thirty and seventy.

That loss of muscle mass can lead to balance problems, trouble walking, slow reaction time (think of catching yourself after you trip or slip), and an increase in fat and, as a result, prediabetes.

But, that doesn't have to happen. Researchers have found that strength training can mitigate age-related declines in how your muscles function. Even just gaining two pounds of muscle can make a huge difference, something that you can do no matter your age.

LESS INFLAMMATION

Maybe you've been hearing about inflammation in recent years as scientists discover just what it can do to the body. Persistent inflammation increases the risk for chronic diseases and can change how your body responds and heals from things like infections, injuries, some cancers, surgeries, and more.

Older adults tend to have elevated levels of inflammation, due to age or age-related issues like being sedentary, which can lead to being overweight or obese. As we get older and experience more issues like arthritis and other joint-related pain, it's harder to move around. As a result, we sit more in order to protect ourselves but, in the end, we end up with higher levels of inflammation and it becomes even harder to move.

Strength training can actually help reduce inflammation, giving you some protection from these concerns.

MORE FLEXIBILITY

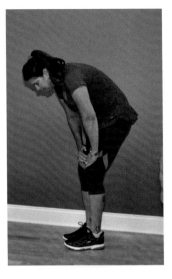

You might not often think about how flexible you are, but tight muscles can have a major effect on how your body functions and feels. You need that flexibility for daily activities such as tying your shoes, reaching for something on a high shelf, folding laundry, or backing out of your driveway.

Flexibility is also important for good posture, circulation, stress, and pain relief (think stretching or yoga), as well as having better balance and the prevention of injuries.

As we age, flexibility naturally declines because our muscles shrink and we lose some muscle fibers. Tendons also lose water content, which is what causes us to feel stiff, especially when we wake up in the morning.

Working on that flexibility, with both stretching and strength training, keeps your body supple, increases flexibility, and increases your range of motion so that everything in life becomes a little easier.

YOUR BRAIN

While exercise and strength training are great for your body and quality of life, you may be surprised at the protective effect exercise can have on your brain.

Here are just some things you can expect to improve with exercise:
- ✓ Prevent or slow mental conditions such as depression, Alzheimer's disease, and Parkinson's disease.
- ✓ Greater amounts of relaxation
  - » Exercise reduces levels of the body's stress hormones while stimulating the production of "feel-good" chemicals in the brain. This means you produce natural painkillers and mood elevators.
- ✓ Improved brain function: Fit seniors are better at processing information more efficiently than seniors who don't exercise.
- ✓ Empowerment
  - » We all feel better about ourselves when we accomplish something, and the feeling of being strong and in control increases confidence and self-efficacy.

✓ Being more integrated into society
  » The stronger you are, the more you can do and the more you'll get out in the world and engage in your community. This alone can contribute even more to those "feel-good" chemicals in the brain, making us feel that we belong.
✓ Better able to adjust to changes
  » Being strong in your body and mind helps you deal with all the changes in your life, retirement, the death of friends or loved ones, health issues, and more.

The bottom line? Exercise is one of the only things you can do for about 10 to 30 minutes a day that can help every part of your brain, cardiovascular system, pulmonary system, sleep, weight management, blood glucose, energy, mood, strength, sex life, and stamina all while helping you feel more confident, empowered, and independent.

Isn't that time much better spent exercising than in a doctor's office? Definitely!

Chapter 3
Getting and Staying Motivated to Exercise

There's no question that exercise is good for us. There is no shortage of evidence that moving more enhances so many aspects of our lives, both physically and psychologically. In fact, many doctors even prescribe it much like they would a pill because they know exercise can:

- ✓ Lower blood pressure
- ✓ Improve sleep
- ✓ Improve your sex life
- ✓ Ease depression and anxiety
- ✓ Improve heart health
- ✓ Help prevent or manage certain types of cancer
- ✓ Increase confidence
- ✓ Help you lose weight and avoid things like diabetes and metabolic syndrome

And of course, there's more that exercise can do for us. The interesting thing is, all of that knowledge doesn't make actually doing the workouts any easier. Just because something is good for us doesn't mean we automatically do it.

We all know that eating lots of fruits and veggies is good for us, but that doesn't mean those are the first things we reach for when we want a snack.

It seems like motivation should just be baked into our bones but, as humans, we are always looking for the easy way out, which means we want to do the least amount of work for the greatest rewards. Makes sense, right?

But exercise can seem like work, which is why many of us avoid it, even knowing the benefits, but there are ways we can use it to our advantage so that it's worth all the effort.

This is where we have to create our own motivation and that often starts with an action rather than a desire.

DIFFERENT TYPES OF MOTIVATION

Motivation comes from a variety of different areas, but we can look at them through two different levels: intrinsic, meaning what comes from inside and extrinsic, which is what drives us from outside ourselves.

INTRINSIC MOTIVATION

One of the ways we motivate ourselves is by having something inside that pushes us to reach outside goals, and often this involves things we enjoy. This could be something we want to accomplish, a competitive edge, or something that will give us pleasure and satisfaction to complete.

For some people exercise is a goal in and of itself. But for others, exercise isn't the end goal we strive for. That doesn't mean we don't want to be healthy, it just means that we want to achieve goals based on our interests, what we enjoy, and what's meaningful to us.

This might mean wanting to be strong for things like gardening, playing with our kids or grandkids, or functioning better when going about the daily activities of life.

Intrinsic goals are ones that motivate from the inside—we strive for something and then we make it happen.

Some exercise-related intrinsic goals might include:

✓ Walking on a regular basis so you can keep up your endurance with your gardening or chores
✓ Playing games with your kids or grandkids for just for fun
✓ Wanting to stay strong to up keep up with your physical hobbies
✓ Wanting to compete in something like a local race for fun and/or charity or a loved one

These are goals we like, that we find interesting, and we get something back from them that is important to us.

Think of someone who gets a diagnosis of breast cancer or some other illness that suddenly changes their lives. This might be the impetus they need to live more healthfully simply because they want to feel better and make a difference in the outcome of their illness.

That kind of internal goal is wonderful and it can drive a variety of behaviors, but it isn't the only way we motivate ourselves. There are other ways to keep us going to reach our goals and, for many of us, those external goals that drive us the most.

EXTRINSIC MOTIVATION

Here's something most of us know, even if we don't want to admit it: Exercise, in and of itself, isn't always a goal we strive for. We know it's good for us. We know we need it . . . but, like choosing broccoli over over macaroni and cheese, it's not always our first choice.

That's where a different type of motivation comes in, the kind that comes from the outside. It's great to have internal goals to drive us, but there are external forces that also motivate us to make a change.

Making use of both of these types of motivation can make regular exercise much more of a reality.

The reality is that most of us rely on a certain amount of extrinsic motivation including:

- ✓ Losing weight
- ✓ Being healthy
- ✓ Making a loved one happy
- ✓ Looking better
- ✓ Meeting new people
- ✓ Fitting into smaller-sized clothing
- ✓ Just feeling good about ourselves

Often it's a mix of intrinsic and extrinsic motivational factors that get us moving and, frankly, it doesn't matter what works... as long as it gets you moving. One day it may be about losing weight and another day it might be about being healthy. Whatever reason you find, it's a good one.

The real key is knowing that you are the one who finds the reason rather than waiting for it to come to you. Most of us don't wake up excited to exercise, right? But most of us will have obstacles in our way. Identifying these obstacles is the first step towards… well, taking that first step.

BARRIERS TO CHANGE

Now we get to the bottom of it, the reasons many of us come up with to avoid exercise and this is an area many of us are very, very good at. Whether you call them "reasons" or "excuses," they typically amount to the same thing—obstacles.

There are plenty of reasons we avoid exercise, and some of them are very good reasons. But, others we can find a way to work around with a little forethought.

FEAR OF INJURY

Fear of hurting yourself is a healthy fear and one that keeps us safe from a variety of injuries in different aspects of life. But then there's exercise, an endeavor that can involve heavy weights and those of us moving them around in different directions, sometimes without any idea what we're doing.

That's where this program can help. Not only do we explain every movement, we teach you how to ease your way into each exercise so you have time to practice and perfect the movement.

There's a built-in learning period where you have time to pay attention to how your body responds to different exercises and adjust accordingly. There are also other things you can do to feel more comfortable:

a. See your doctor: You hear this all the time from commercials, but that is literally what your doctor is there for. If you have any concerns, write them down and ask about each one. It's okay to be fully invested in your health and walk into an exercise program with confidence.
b. Err on the side of caution: If you're not sure about something, skip it. I've worked with a variety of clients and if they feel anything strange about

what they're doing, we stop. There are so many exercises out there, there is always a substitution.

    c.   Listen to your body: I say this a lot to clients, but it bears repeating. No one knows your body better than you. While you don't want to be so cautious that you don't try anything new, there's a middle ground to shoot for.

As always, if you question anything, stop. There's always another day.

ISN'T IT "NO PAIN, NO GAIN"?

One theory many of us grew up with was without pain, there is no gain. That's definitely outdated thinking, born more from the bodybuilding age than our current one.

What we've learned over time is that, first, our definition of pain isn't the same as it used to be. If you think of the older times of aerobics, bodybuilding, and more, somehow having an injury was a badge of honor.

I remember training clients who would throw up in a trash can, thinking that was what "real" exercise was.

Now, we know a lot more than we did back then and we know we don't have to push our limits that far to get results.

The second part of that is this question: Is pain really the threshold we want to achieve with exercise? Maybe if you're competing in the Olympics or some mega-important race.

But what if we're just trying to get stronger? Maybe lose some weight? Maybe we just want to feel good in our bodies.

Perhaps pain isn't what we're looking for to reach our goal, and here's something I want all my clients to remember: Exercise does not have to hurt.

Is there some exertion? Of course. If you want to make big changes in your body, that definitely means big changes in how you work that body as well as how you feed it and care for it.

But for those of us who simply want to be strong in the bodies we have, we may already be in pain. For many of us, we're dealing with ongoing issues such as arthritis, old injuries that flare up when it rains, and previous surgeries that left us a little less symmetrical than we once were.

That's where listening to your body comes in. Yes, there is always some kind of effort, maybe a level of discomfort that comes with working out, but it shouldn't be more than that.

It's good to be vigilant and pay attention to how you feel. That will keep you focused on what works for your body and what doesn't, without being afraid to try new things.

Our goal now is no pain. At all.

DEALING WITH ONGOING PHYSICAL ISSUES AND CONDITIONS

It's rare that any of us make it to our later years without having some wear and tear and things that can get in the way of maintaining mobility. It's this type of situation that can give you the most problems because you don't want to exacerbate an ongoing issue.

This kind of thing is best dealt with your doctor and/or a physical therapist, but some very basic advice I give my clients:

✓ Find a workaround— Even if you can't, say, work your lower body, you can still work your upper body from a seated position. In fact, you'll find a variety of seated exercises in this book. Feel free to cherry-pick the moves that work for your body, however it is right now.

✓ Get professional advice— Any time an old injury flares up, this is the time to talk to your doctor or maybe get a referral to a physical therapist. Sometimes you want to know what to avoid to exacerbate the problem, something that should come from a professional.

✓ Do what you can—We've all had old conditions flare up and, sometimes it's just a matter of doing whatever you can to stay moving. Maybe that's just taking a short daily walk, doing some simple stretches, or just walking around the house. It all counts.

The goal is to keep moving in whatever form that looks like. Maybe you do everything seated or using no weights. Feel free to create something that fits where you are. And if you're not sure, it's okay to ask for help, whether that's from a personal trainer, a physical therapist, or a doctor.

CONFUSION OVER HOW TO START

As simple as exercise seems, when you try to actually get started, it gets very confusing. What exercises do you do? How many? How do you know you're doing it right?

There's no end to the information out there about exercise, but this book puts all the guidelines together so you don't have to worry if you're doing it right.

Too many of us make exercise more complicated than it has to be and, yes, strength training does have a learning curve. But, everything you need to succeed is here, including:

- ✓ Specific exercises and workouts—The workouts here are mapped out according to science and what we personal trainers have come to learn is the best way to start. Your only goal is to try each exercise, determine which ones work for you, and use your best form for each exercise. Over time, you'll learn much more about your body and be able to expand from these exercises.
- ✓ A schedule to follow—The other thing that throws us off is figuring when and how to exercise, something this program helps you with. You'll get a suggested schedule every two weeks, but you can easily adjust it to fit with your personal schedule and how you feel. You'll have instructions for how to adapt this program to fit your personal schedule and needs.
- ✓ Rest days—Rest days are built into the program but, of course, you're in charge of when you need rest, giving you full control over your program.
- ✓ Suggested weights—Choosing weights can be one of the more challenging aspects of lifting weights, and there isn't always a great way to teach that without being there in your living room. The suggested weights in this program give you a place to start, and you can always switch weights whenever something feels too heavy or too light.

TIME CONSTRAINTS

The other reason many of us skip exercise is because we're just too busy. Life is full of things we have to do. If you made a to-do list right now, it would probably list more things than you could even do in one day.

I have that same to-do list.

Here's news that many of my clients don't like to hear: Exercisers are no less busy than the average person. In fact, they actually have the same number of hours in a day that the rest of us have.

If that doesn't make you feel any better about yourself, you're not alone.

The real key is:

Prioritizing.

It's more about prioritizing your time than needing more of it (which, goodness knows, we'd love to be able to have), and there are some things you can do to make exercise more of a priority on your list:

a. Remember your goals: This is time-worn advice, I know, but there is something very powerful about having your goals right in front of you on a daily basis. Write them down. Put them on sticky notes and place them on your computer, your wall, your steering wheel. I have a process where I put my goals on sticky notes and, every time I reach one, I move that note to a different wall. Every day I can actually see what I've accomplished. Try this method and see if it works for you.

b. Schedule it: This isn't the first time you've heard this and it won't be the last. I don't know about your life, but when I don't schedule something it simply doesn't get done. Take some time at the beginning of the week to schedule your appointments, including your workouts, so there are no excuses. Write it down, type it in, however you keep your calendar. Do it at the beginning of the week so it's there in the front of your mind.

c. Do it at the same time: There's not a "right" time to exercise. Some of us prefer early while others like the afternoon. Whatever your preference, schedule it at the same time. Your body will often instigate your workout before your mind even knows what's happening. It's like brushing your teeth—it becomes automatic even if you don't feel like it.

d. Involve other activities or family members: Make your workouts more fun by involving other family members or doing things outside in the fresh air. It doesn't always have to be inside with equipment. Plan a regular walk after lunch or dinner, something that becomes a part of your regular routine.

And don't forget, there are things built into us that make us want to change, and harnessing those can make it that much easier. That's where having clear goals can really make a difference.

WHAT MOTIVATES US TO MAKE A CHANGE?

You've learned about motivation, the kind that drives us from the inside and the outside, but there are some specific things that have the most impact on us.

As we get older and want to participate in life, there's one area we all want to improve: Health. In fact, it's the one thing wasted on the young, right? You don't know what's going to happen to your body as you age until it does. And, boy, does it.

Health often becomes one of the main reasons we decide to make a change, and it's easy to see why.

IMPROVING HEALTH

Improving health can be a big motivator depending on a person's situation. Maybe it's that first time your doctor put you on a medication you never thought you'd need. Maybe it's having that surgery you weren't planning on. Either way, things will happen to derail you from basic life tasks including:

- ✓ Pain—Pain is a definite motivator, something anyone who's been through a major injury, surgery, etc. can tell you. Being in pain changes how you act, how you feel, and what you do to deal with it. For many, it's a reason to get stronger so as to avoid it.
- ✓ Getting off certain kinds of medication—Some medications are necessary, but there are others we might be able to wean off of with exercise. High blood pressure, diabetic medication, or even anti-depressants are things that, in theory, we can manage with lifestyle changes. Obviously this should be done through the purview of your doctor.
- ✓ Better sleep—One thing we often notice as we get older is that sleep is harder to come by and most of us know the benefits of getting enough sleep including reducing stress, weight loss, and allowing our bodies to rest and rejuvenate. Numerous studies show that regular exercise can

increase the amount of slow wave sleep we get, the kind that helps us get the rest we need.

✓ More energy—Science has shown that an object at rest tends to stay at rest. But an object in motion? Yes... stays in motion. The more you move, the more energy you generate, and exercise has been proven to enhance those "feel-good" hormones such as endorphins, hormones designed to boost our moods and make us feel better.

✓ More clarity—If there's one thing movement can do, it's to allow us time to let the mind wander a bit and that often brings clarity to regular, everyday problems we might chew over, given a little too much time inside our minds. Giving your mind a break with some mindless exercise may help you solve problems a little easier.

SELF-EFFICACY

One of the most important ways we feel motivated is by taking on a challenge and then conquering that challenge. No doubt you've experienced any number of challenging situations and one thing we learn is that we can always do more than we think.

That's where self-efficacy comes in. Self-efficacy sounds like a fancy word, but it really refers to the fact that you have complete confidence in your abilities. Whether that's confidence in your own motivation or over your own environment, that belief is what adds to your ability to control what's going on around you.

Part of this confidence comes through practice. Every time you show up for a workout, every time you reach for a pair of weights, you increase your own sense of belief in yourself. It really is all about believing in your own capacity to do this. And that happens every time you show up.

There are different ways we can experience self-efficacy including:

a. Experience: Mastering any task, even if it's mastering an exercise program, gives you that achievement that helps you keep going. It's like gardening. When I started out, I had no idea what I was doing (sometimes still don't). But over time, I've learned a lot just by trying and that makes me want to do more.

b. Modeling: This may involve having someone in your life who's succeeding at something. For example, my husband started walking regularly and, just seeing him do that was motivating enough for me to realize I could do it too. Looking around at the people in your life can give you inspiration to make a change.

c. Social persuasion: This type of motivation can come from someone you know or, in some cases, belonging to a group. Whether that's a gym or some other like-minded people, seeing those people or being invited to join them can also be a motivator to help you master different tasks.

BELIEVING WE CAN SUCCEED

One important part of this mix is believing in ourselves, especially during difficult situations. Some of us are going through a variety of issues: back problems, arthritis, joint issues, and other things that cause chronic pain.

One of the most important things that keeps us going is knowing we can succeed. What keeps us from believing that? Fear.

Part of believing in ourselves is dealing with the fear that all of us feel from time to time. Fear of failure.

OVERCOMING FEAR OF FAILURE

Is it really possible to completely overcome fear of failure? I don't think so, although working on it is certainly a worthwhile venture. Fear serves a very important purpose in our lives, knowing when to avoid something that may harm us being just one.

When it comes to exercise, fear of failure tops the list of reasons to avoid it. While we're all born with the same knowledge, there's some part of us that believes we are just born knowing how to exercise.

It's that belief that has us walking into gyms thinking that we're just supposed to know how all these contraptions work and exactly how to use them.

The good news is that no one is born knowing these things and, second, you can learn at your own pace and make decisions that work for your body.

The truth is that some days, you will fail. As humans, it's what we do, but that doesn't mean we give up. One way to deal with that failure is to:

- ✓ Set goals based on what you know you can reach—Here's the good news: You don't have to have the same goals day after day. Sometimes what we can accomplish changes based on how we feel from day to day. Sometimes, it's the best decision to change your goal rather than force something that just isn't going to happen through no fault of your own.
- ✓ Focus on the energy you need for now—Too often we think of exercise as something we have to do day after day after day. In reality, we only need enough energy for what we need to do right now. Tomorrow's energy will come and then we can rely on that.
- ✓ Be okay with what you can do—Every day is different. Some days you knock it out of the park and others you're just happy you made it out of bed. Celebrate what you can do each day and adjust for that difference. It's normal and it's okay.

FINDING SOCIAL SUPPORT

One of the most important coping strategies when it comes to exercise is developing strong social support. Having a social network, whether it's online or local, is one way to keep that belief that you can succeed.

The great thing about current times is that there are many ways to stay social, even if you're at home and don't always have the means to meet other people.

- ✓ Meetups (https://www.meetup.com/) are one of the best ways to find people who are into what you're into. This free website allows you to sign up and join groups that match your interests, whether that's hiking, biking, dancing, or book clubs.
- ✓ Nextdoor (https://nextdoor.com/news_feed/) is a great way to keep up with what's going on locally and reach out when you need help with almost anything.
- ✓ Community resources: Your next best bet is to use community resources to find out what's going on in your neighborhood. Your local library or community center often has a variety of groups and gatherings that may meet your needs.

Chapter 4
What You Need to Know to Get Started

Before you start any kind of exercise program or meal plan, there are things you can do to prepare and make sure you're ready for what's to come. These steps can give you the confidence to get started, knowing you're stepping out on the right foot.

1. Do I Need to See a Doctor First?

If you haven't seen a doctor or had a physical in a while, I highly recommend you get one, whether you're exercising or not.

Getting a baseline for everything from your weight to your blood pressure keeps you up-to-date on what's going on with your body, and these baselines can also be used as a measuring tool to see how you progress.

As you start exercising, you may notice changes in your blood pressure, weight, resting heart rate, and more. This is just one way to track your progress and see how exercise affects your health overall.

Beyond that, there are definitely times you should see your doctor before doing any kind of exercise:

- ✓ If you're on certain medications that can affect your heart rate during exercise or other aspects of movement. The most common medications that may change how your body responds to exercise include:
  - » Blood pressure medications
  - » Antidepressants
  - » Antihistamines
  - » Diabetes medications

» Heart medication
» Diuretics

If you're not sure, or if any of the following scenarios apply, call your doctor to find out what you need to know about your medications and exercise.

✓ You have a chronic illness, injury, or medical condition like heart disease, kidney disease, diabetes, or arthritis, just to name a few. You want to talk to your doctor about what you should or, more importantly, shouldn't do that might aggravate your condition.
✓ You're worried about a past injury or condition and want to make sure your body is ready for exercise.
✓ You've had a recent illness or surgery.

2. Proper Clothes and Footwear

You don't have to have anything fancy to start working out, but you want to be comfortable and you want your body to be supported by the right kind of shoes.

For your workout clothes, focus on:

✓ **Loose-fitting, comfortable clothes:** Sweatpants, shorts, tights, and T-shirts are all fine for exercise, as long as they're not so loose that they get in the way.
✓ **Sweat-wicking clothes:** There are a lot of companies out there making sweat-wicking fitness gear from shirts and tights to socks and sports bras. You can definitely opt for these if you find cotton uncomfortable or you find you're sweating a lot (cotton gets very heavy with sweat). You can find very affordable exercise wear at places such as TJ Maxx, Target, Walmart, and other department stores.

You want to make sure your body is fully supported, so shoes are very important. But there are hundreds of shoes out there for all kinds of foot structures, arches, and more. If you can, try going to a specialty store (usually a running or walking store) and have your feet measured and your arches checked to find the right shoe for you. This is the least confusing way to get a great pair of shoes.

If that's not an option and you're at a department store or shopping online, focus on these areas:

- ✓ **Motion control:** This refers to the amount of stability your shoes offer when you're walking or working out. A stable shoe will support your ankles and arches.
- ✓ **Breathable and lightweight:** When trying on shoes, notice the difference between materials and comfort. You don't want the shoes to feel stiff and tight. You should be able to walk in them right away without breaking them in.
- ✓ **Cushioning and support:** Make sure to walk in the shoes you're checking out to check for support. Good support will ensure that there's less stress on your feet and legs.

I always tell my clients to spend the most money on shoes, since they are the literal foundation of everything you're going to be doing. If budget is an issue, you can always get fitted for a shoe and then shop online to find it for a lower price.

3. What Equipment Do You Need, and Where Do You Get It?

For the majority of the workouts, we'll be doing bodyweight exercises and using simple equipment like weights and bands.

Here's what you need for all the workouts you'll be doing in the next twelve weeks.

- a. **A variety of dumbbells:** If you're new to strength training and don't have any weights, I recommend you start with about three or four sets of dumbbells. Think of it as having a light, medium, and heavy set of dumbbells. Here are some general suggestions, but you'll be more apt to pick the right amount of weight with some experimentation and practice:
  - i. For women, light: 2 to 5 pounds, medium: 5 to 8 pounds, heavy: 8 to 10 pounds.
  - ii. For men, light: 5 to 8 pounds, medium: 8 to 10 pounds, Heavy: 10 to 12 pounds.

iii. You can get the best deals on weights at discount department stores (Walmart, Target, etc.) or at places like Play It Again Sports. You can even check around at garage sales. You'll almost always find something exercise related that sat in someone's basement for years. But you're not going to have that problem, right?

b. **Resistance bands:** I love resistance bands for working the body in a different way than dumbbells. Unlike weights, bands have tension during the lifting and lower phase of an exercise, so you target even more muscles. Bands come in a variety of tensions and colors, so don't let that confuse you. You can buy them at sporting goods stores or places like Target or Walmart. I recommend getting at least two bands because they have different levels of tension. My preferred bands come from my favorite company, SPRI. Here's what I use in my home gym (these can be ordered at Spri.com or amazon.com):
   i. Light tension: SPRI Deluxe Xertub Resistance Band Color **Yellow**
   ii. Medium tension: SPRI Deluxe Xertub Resistance Band Color **Green**
   iii. Heavy tension: SPRI Deluxe Xertub Resistance Band Color **Red**

c. **Gliding/sliding devices**: Now, this may sound a little crazy if you haven't heard of these, but gliding exercises are an excellent tool for hitting all kinds of fitness goals like cardio, strength, balance, stability, and even flexibility. You basically put a foot or hand on the disc and go through a variety of sliding moves. There are different tools you can use for gliding exercises, which include:
   i. **Gliding discs:** These are made by, er, Gliding Discs! You can order these from amazon.com. Just search for "gliding discs" and look for the purple ones made by Gliding Discs. They come in two different varieties, one set for carpet (these are slippery and slide easily on carpet) or one set for hardwood floors (these are made of different material).

ii. **Towels:** If you have hardwood floors you can use small towels, but be careful. Sometimes they can slide fast so you want to feel safe using them.

iii. **Paper plates:** If you have carpet, you can try paper plates to slide but, again, you get what you pay for. It kind of depends on your carpet.

SETTING YOUR GOALS

A big part of starting an exercise program is to have some goals for what you want to accomplish. It's great to have broad goals such as getting healthy, getting stronger, or losing weight, but you have to get specific. Otherwise, how do you know if you're reaching your goals?

That's why it's important to set S.M.A.R.T. goals.

That means your goals should be

- ✓ **Specific**—Maybe your goal is to improve your balance, but what does that actually look like? Being able to stand on one foot while putting on your socks? Maybe it means feeling more confident when you're walking down the stairs. Be specific about exactly what you want to achieve.
- ✓ **Measurable**—The next important part of setting goals is making sure you can measure them. If you want to lose weight, you can measure that on a scale, but what if you want some other goal that isn't so cut and dried? Maybe a good goal would be doing a certain number of workouts a week, which you can easily measure.
- ✓ **Attainable**—It's great to have long-term goals, but think of the short-term. What can you actually do right now? Maybe you'd like to work out five days a week, but a more achievable goal might be two or three days a week to start. Maybe your goal is even one workout a week. The more successful you are, the more you'll stick to your goals.
- ✓ **Relevant**—This is related to setting specific goals in that you want this to be something that matters to you right now. Maybe losing weight is a

goal, but what you really need to focus on is feeling stronger and more independent. Set a goal that means improving your life.

✓ **Time-bound**—The last aspect of setting goals is to have some kind of timeline to achieve it. This program gives you twelve weeks of strength training workouts, so that's a great timeline to start off with.

Setting goals that are too vague (i.e., I'll walk twice this week) are easy to put off. But, if you decide you're going to walk on Mondays and Wednesdays at 8:30 a.m. at the local mall, it's much easier to stick to it.

TRACKING YOUR PROGRESS

The only way to know if you're actually getting somewhere with your exercise program is to regularly track your progress. You can easily make your own workout log by simply writing down the exercises each week and noting how much weight you use each time and how each exercise feels.

You can record your workouts, weights used, etc. but you can also track things in other ways.

A simple calendar on the wall can give you a visual of your progress. By marking off the days you work out, you can see how you're doing and if you're showing up for your workouts on a consistent basis.

Keeping a basic health and fitness journal can also help. For example, if you miss some workouts, you can figure out what went wrong, if anything, and you can keep a general record of how you're feeling and doing. It may be you missed a workout because you were sore, which might mean you need more recovery time.

You can find a variety of free fitness tracking worksheets to download on the Internet, or just keep a pad and pen handy whenever you work out.

There are also online and smartphone tools to help you track your progress, many of which are free. One is My Fitness Pal, https://www.myfitnesspal.com/, which is free and allows you to track everything from your computer or smartphone app. You can track your diet, exercise, nutrients, and you can even scan barcodes of food to find the nutrient content of different foods.

FitWatch, https://www.fitwatch.com/, is another free website where you can find trackers, calculators, and much more about health and fitness.

Choose a system that works for you and make it a habit to log what you're doing on a daily basis. Seeing and appreciating your progress is a powerful thing.

FALLING OFF THE WAGON—NOW WHAT?

It's inevitable that life will happen, and sometimes that interferes with your workouts. There are a variety of things that happen to throw us off track, many of them unexpected.

- ✓ An illness
- ✓ An injury
- ✓ A life change such as changing jobs, getting married, losing someone close to us
- ✓ Moving
- ✓ Time or family commitments
- ✓ The weather
- ✓ Boredom
- ✓ Fatigue

The list goes on, and it's important to recognize that this is normal and to be realistic about what you can and can't do. We can't be perfect all the time, but the key is to get back to your workouts as soon as you can.

Even taking just one small action can get you back into your exercise groove. Try simple things like taking walks, doing the warm-up exercises instead of an entire workout, or taking a few extra stairs throughout the day.

We all get off track for one reason or another, but there's no reason you can't get back on track. You just have to do one positive thing in that direction and you'll find your momentum again.

ADVICE ON CHOOSING YOUR WEIGHTS

While I offer suggestions for the amount of weight to use for different exercises, it's important to know that what you use is different for everyone.

Experts typically use a percentage of your one repetition maximum, meaning you lift as much as you can for one repetition of an exercise, say a biceps curl, and then use a percentage of that to figure out how much weight you need for more reps.

For most of us, lifting a very heavy weight one time isn't safe or feasible. It's much better to choose a weight to lift for the suggested repetitions and then pay attention to your body's signals.

Let's say you're doing an exercise for ten repetitions, which is typical of many exercises. If you get to the tenth repetition and you feel like you could do a lot more, that's a good sign you could go heavier.

If you can't finish all the repetitions without losing your form, that means you may need to go down in weight.

Keep in mind that every day is different. Some days you're feeling energetic and may be able to do more and other days maybe not.

Your tracking forms can help you keep track of the weights you're using and how they feel to you.

One other thing to think about is that, if you're a beginner, you're going to get results with just about any amount of resistance. Any new challenge you add to your body will stimulate that muscle growth, especially if you're just starting out.

It's much better to focus on your form and doing the exercises correctly than it is to worry about how much weight you're lifting.

DELAYED ONSET MUSCLE SORENESS (DOMS) AND REST DAYS

One other important aspect to consider is soreness. It's very normal to get sore after doing any new activity, including exercise and strength training.

This program is designed to ease you into strength training so that you can progress gradually, which can help with soreness. However, some stiffness should be expected. The only way our muscles grow is when we give them more than they can handle.

When we do that, our muscles respond by adapting and growing more muscle fibers. That's part of the delayed onset muscle soreness (DOMS) we often experience within two or three days after a new activity.

Think of when you first do yard work after a long season and how your body feels the next day. Anything you haven't done in a while has the potential to leave you sore and tired, and the same can be true of resistance training.

SYMPTOMS OF DOMS

- ✓ Your muscles may feel tender to the touch
- ✓ You may feel stiffness and soreness when you move, especially after you've been sitting for a while
- ✓ Some swelling in the muscles
- ✓ Muscle fatigue

It's normal to feel some burning while doing the exercises, which is a sign your muscles are working. That should go away when you finish the exercise. DOMS is different in that it usually takes about twelve hours before it shows up, although many people find that forty-eight hours after the workout is the most painful.

WHAT TO DO ABOUT DOMS

Some soreness is to be expected and, for the most part, time is your best bet.

There are other solutions you can try.

- ✓ Take an over-the-counter painkiller such as ibuprofen (make sure you talk to your doctor first about any other medications you're on)
- ✓ Try using a muscle relief cream such as Bengay or Sombra
- ✓ Take a hot bath or shower
- ✓ Get a massage

It's also a good idea to keep moving, even if you're sore. Keeping your muscles warm will help you feel better, even if it doesn't speed up the healing process. Keep in mind that, if you can barely move after a workout, you likely overdid it and should back off on your weights and workouts.

REST DAYS

Rest is just as important as your workout. It's only during the rest days that your muscles grow. Your workout is the stimulus, and your body responds during recovery periods.

A rest day doesn't necessarily mean you sit around doing nothing. In fact, doing some movement will actually help you make progress. Your body needs circulation to bring nutrients to your muscles, so movement actually helps the process.

How much rest you need is based on a number of factors including fitness level, age, other activities you may be involved in, sleep habits, and more.

In this program, you'll have scheduled rest days, but it's important to know what works for you. If you're very sore, consider taking an extra day or two off from exercise and get back to it when the soreness is gone.

The last thing you want is to overdo it and end up with a longer recovery period, although it's usually okay to do some light movement if you're feeling stiff rather than sore.

Doing some light cardio on rest days is a great way to stay active and keep the blood moving in your body.

PAIN VS. DISCOMFORT

You've probably heard plenty of sayings about exercise like, "No pain, no gain." But, in the world of fitness there's a big difference between the effort it takes to lift weights and actual pain.

Yes, your muscles may burn as you're lifting weights during the exercise, and that's a normal feeling that should go away when you stop. But pain during an exercise is entirely different and a sign that you may be doing a movement your body just doesn't like.

If you feel any sharp pains in your joints during an exercise, that's a sign to stop and either change how you're doing the move or skip it completely.

Other issues to watch out for is chronic pain, such as tendinitis, which you may feel during the workout and after. This could be due to an overuse injury or some other condition, and you should check with your doctor before you keep exercising.

If anything doesn't feel right, err on the side of caution and stop what you're doing. It may take some time to get used to the exercises before you know what's normal discomfort and what's an injury or situation that may require a doctor's attention.

Chapter 5
Exercise Guidelines for Seniors

Now, you know that the government and other entities like to tell us just how much exercise we need to be healthy, lose weight, etc. Seniors are no exception, but trying to actually follow these "rules" and adapt them to your life can be downright confusing.

The Office of Disease Prevention and Health Promotion (ODPHP) regularly updates the Physical Activity Guidelines for Americans, grouping it according to age and fitness level. You can find the full guidelines at https://health.gov/paguidelines/second-edition/.

I'm going to break it down so you know what the guidelines are and then how to adapt those guidelines for your particular situation. Every person varies, and we're all starting from different places.

The guidelines are just that, a rough outline of what to shoot for, not rules that you *must* follow. Remember, this is your body and you know it better than anyone else, so never be afraid to adjust anything that doesn't feel good.

In addition, the guidelines don't always address each person's fitness level. For example, the general recommendations below suggest 2.5 to 5 hours a week of exercise. That may be a good timeline to shoot for if you've been working out for a while but, if you're new, you might need to start with 10 minutes a day and work your way up.

General Exercise Guidelines for Older Adults	
General exercise recommendations	✓ 150 to 300 minutes (2.5 to 5 hours) per week unless you have physical conditions that may hamper your ability to exercise, in which case do as much as you can to avoid being sedentary
Cardio exercise such as walking, swimming, or cycling	✓ Experts recommend you do cardio about 3 days a week at a moderate intensity or, if you're a regular exerciser, you can mix moderate intensity (level 5 on a scale of 1 to 10) and vigorous-intensity workouts (level 7 or 8 on a scale of 1 to 10)
Strength training	✓ Exercises that work all the major muscle groups at least 2 times a week
Flexibility training	✓ Doing regular flexibility exercises at least 2 to 3 times a week allows your joints to move more freely through a full range of motion, thus reducing your chances of injuries

Let's break down these guidelines into what it would look like in real life.

CARDIO EXERCISE

While we'll focus more on strength training throughout the book, cardio exercise is another important part of getting stronger and being able to do more in your life. You may think that cardio involves high-impact activities such as running, jumping, or high-intensity interval training, but at its most basic, cardio exercise is simply any rhythmic movement you do for an extended period of time.

Here are just some of the activities you have to choose from:

✓ Walking
✓ Jogging
✓ Running
✓ Tennis
✓ Pickleball
✓ Basketball

- ✓ Swimming
- ✓ Cycling
- ✓ Vigorous yard work or housework (think raking leaves or mopping the floor)
- ✓ Hiking
- ✓ Active yoga (vinyasa or power yoga)
- ✓ Dancing
- ✓ Exercise classes (aerobics, kickboxing, etc.)

Even chasing the kids or grandkids or tossing a ball in the backyard can count as cardio exercise.

The idea with cardio is to work just a bit out of your comfort zone, depending on your fitness level.

Think of a scale of 1 to 10, like the one below:

Perceived Exertion Chart

Level 1: I'm lounging around watching TV and feeling great.

Level 2: I'm moving around a little and feel just fine.

Level 3: I'm taking a leisurely stroll or puttering around and could probably do this all day.

Level 4: I'm moving faster now and I might even start sweating soon. This is starting to feel suspiciously like exercise.

Level 5: Now I know I'm exercising, but I'm only a little out of my comfort zone. I can still talk and I'm okay.

Level 6: I'm working harder now and can still talk, but it's becoming more difficult. I'm totally exercising now.

Level 7: Okay, now I'm breathing harder and I can talk, but only in short sentences.

Level 8: I'm working really hard and can only stay at this level for a short time. I could huff out a word or two if forced.

Level 9: I cannot talk. At all. I think I might be dying.

Level 10: I am dead.

Obviously this is a little tongue in cheek and not an official version of a perceived exertion chart, but it gives you an idea of how the exercise feels to you and what level of intensity you're at. You generally want to shoot for around level 5 or 6 for a moderate-intensity workout.

For example, say you're going for a walk. To get to a level 5, pretend that you're walking fast to catch a bus that's in the distance, but you don't want to break into a run because you have a bad knee. That's getting you just out of your comfort zone, but not so far that you hate what you're doing.

More advanced exercisers can opt for higher intensity like speed walking, running, or high-intensity interval training, which would get you around level 7 or 8, maybe even 9 depending on what you're doing.

The point is, this kind of exercise makes your heart strong, increases your stamina and endurance, and it also burns calories, a plus if you want to lose a few pounds.

If you're a beginner or it's been a bit since you've exercised, you might start with a light walking workout two to three times a week at a low to moderate pace. Start with 5 or 10 minutes and slowly increase your walking time as you get stronger and fitter.

Now, the guidelines suggest 150 to 300 minutes, which would come out to about twenty to forty minutes a day, but start with what feels good to you. Even five minutes counts.

STRENGTH TRAINING

Now we get into the nitty-gritty of what you'll be doing in the 12-week program. To start, we'll do a quick overview of the guidelines for strength training to give you an idea of what's to come.

I've talked about the benefits of strength training, but what do you do and how often? This program will show you exactly that, but the ODPHP has some basics to get you started.

The idea with strength training is to make your muscles do more work than they're used to doing. You've probably experienced this a number of times, like whenever the seasons change and you do something you haven't done in months such as gardening or shoveling snow.

You're overloading your muscles which, in the short-term, can cause some muscle soreness but, in the long-term, leads to building lean muscle tissue.

Here are some general guidelines:

- ✓ Muscle-strengthening activities include lifting weights, using resistance bands, bodyweight exercises, heavy gardening, or even carrying heavy loads on a regular basis.
- ✓ For the most benefit, you should focus on working the major muscle groups which include the chest, back, shoulders, biceps, triceps, lower body, and core.
- ✓ You should aim to lift weights on at least two non-consecutive days a week.
- ✓ For each exercise, you want to do between 8 and 16 repetitions for about one to three sets. Repetitions refer to the number of times you do an exercise and a set refers to how many times you do that exercise consecutively. For example, if you lift and lower a weight 10 times, you've completed ten reps in one set. You'll see this throughout the program expressed as the number of sets times the reps, such as 1 x 10 (one set of ten reps).
- ✓ You should increase the amount of weight as you get stronger and you can also add another day of strength training as well.

You'll learn more about all of this throughout the rest of the book and find specifics about how to manipulate different elements of your strength training workouts once the program ends. These principles will guide you in continuing to progress long after the program is over.

FLEXIBILITY TRAINING

Another piece of the puzzle is flexibility, something that tends to decline as we age. That's usually because our muscles shrink naturally, which may reduce our range of motion.

Flexibility is all about the range of motion within your joints. One great example is your hip joint. If you can imagine lifting your right knee straight up to your hip, then circling that knee to the right, that gives you an idea of range of motion.

But there are a number of things that can contribute to lack of range of motion such as:

- ✓ Genes—Some us of are more flexible simply because we've inherited that gene
- ✓ Joint structure—One thing we can't control is the actual structure of our joints, which may limit our range of motion
- ✓ Connective tissue—Things like ligaments, tendons, and muscles can make a difference in how your joints move and how flexible you are
- ✓ Strength—One other important part is the strength of your opposing muscles. That means the muscles that are opposite from one another such as your biceps are opposing muscles to your triceps. Here's an example: If your quadriceps (on the front of the legs) are tight, that could hinder the flexibility of your hamstrings, on the back of the legs. So working on flexibility on both sides of the body can help

The bottom line is that working on flexibility, as you will in this program, will help minimize some of the factors that contribute to balance issues. The other important part of working on range of motion exercises is that these moves can increase the synovial fluid to your joints. This allows a greater freedom of movement and also may decelerate the degeneration of the joints.

BALANCE TRAINING

Fall prevention is one of the most important things to conquer for all of us, especially older adults. The statistics can be eye-opening. The National Council on Aging has found that:

- ✓ Falls are the leading cause of fatal and non-fatal injuries for older adults
- ✓ Falls result in more than 2.8 million injuries each year
- ✓ The cost of injuries caused by falls was more than $50 billion in 2015

The emotional and psychological cost of falling, or even just fear of falling, has an enormous impact on older adults. A growing number of older adults are afraid of falling and, as a result, limit their activities, which only adds to a further decline in physical ability.

Limiting activities has much more impact than just physically. When you're afraid of falling or even getting in and out of a car, you might stay home more, which can lead to to social isolation, depression, and feelings of helplessness.

Here's what's important to know: Falling is not inevitable just because we get older. In fact, we have some level of control over that by how we exercise and take care of our bodies, which is an important part of this 12-week program.

Balance problems are one reason many adults seek help from a doctor because that lack of balance affects almost every aspect of life such as:

- ✓ Walking without staggering or falling
- ✓ Getting up and down from a chair without falling
- ✓ Climbing stairs without tripping
- ✓ Bending over without falling

Good balance is so important for staying healthy and maintaining independence, which is why it's critical to incorporate balance exercises into your daily life.

Balance issues can have a number of causes, so you should talk to your doctor about to try to identify the impetus. Just a few issues include high blood pressure, ear infection, stroke, or multiple sclerosis.

Barring those issues, if you don't have any other conditions, balance training can become a very important part of your daily activity. Balance focuses on those smaller areas we don't often think about such as the tendons and ligaments that hold our joints together.

There are also very small muscles that work to help stabilize us. The muscles of the feet, the ankles, and the knees are crucial to keeping us mobile and healthy. The balance exercises in this book will help you work on all of these areas in a safe environment that will help you improve so that you can stay strong and independent.

CORE TRAINING

Another very important part of aging in a healthy way is to give your body a strong foundation to work from. That foundation is your core. Think of your core, which is comprised of much more than your abs, as the sun around which your body revolves. The stronger and brighter it is, the stronger and brighter the rest of your body is as well.

So, what is the core?

We often think the core just includes the abs, but it actually includes not just the outer abs but the underlying muscles as well. These include:

- ✓ The rectus abdominis—If you've ever heard of the "six-pack" muscles, then you've heard of the rectus abdominis. These muscles are responsible for bending your torso forward, as when you do a crunch.
- ✓ The transverse abdominis—This is like a secret muscle under the rectus abdominis that wraps around your spine. If you can imagine someone about to punch you, this is the muscle that contracts to protect you and your spine. When you do a plank (which you will do in this program), that's the muscle you're strengthening.
- ✓ The obliques—The internal and external obliques are on either side of your waist and help you twist as well as bend to either side. They're often described as "pockets" you can slide your hands into to move your torso in the right direction.
- ✓ The erector spinae—This is a fancy word for the small muscles of your back that travel down either side of the spine. These muscles are responsible for helping you bend and straighten as well as bend backwards. If you ever do housework or gardening, you've definitely felt these muscles.

These are all the muscle groups that create the powerhouse of your body and serve as the origin from which many movements come. An important part of your workouts involve core stabilization so that you can hold the spine in the right position while you move other parts of the body.

The great thing about strengthening the core is that there are multiple ways to do that, not just doing exercises on the floor like crunches, which most of us have done at one time or another.

In this program, you'll do targeted core work as well as general strength training, which also involves your core in a more functional way, supporting your body through a variety of movements, just like real life.

All of these things together—strength training, balance training, core training, and flexibility work—all help you build a stronger, more resilient body for whatever you might encounter.

FOCUSING ON FORM

One more very important part of the picture is having good form when doing your exercises. In fact, your form is far more important than any other part of your workout, but what does that mean?

Every exercise is different and you'll have instructions for each one, but there are some basics to follow no matter what you're doing.

- ✓ Good posture: Whether you're sitting or standing, you want to begin each exercise with good posture. That includes:
  - » Sitting or standing tall as though your head is attached to a string pulling you up towards the ceiling.
  - » If you're standing, take the feet about hip-width apart and keep a slight bend in the knees to have a strong foundation from which to move.
- ✓ A strong core: As mentioned, core stabilization is an important part of every exercise you do. Almost all the movements you make originate from your torso, which includes your abs, back, and pelvic area. Keeping a strong core means that you brace your abs before you do any type of movement. This gives you the support you need for the exercises to come, protecting you from injury and giving you the most out of the movement. Not only that, but a strong core helps you keep your balance, something that will be a big help in the balancing exercises.
- ✓ Focusing on the movement: Each exercise targets a particular muscle group, although other muscle groups are often involved. In general, you want to focus your attention on the muscles you're working and avoid swinging the weights or using momentum to lift the weights.
- ✓ Protecting your joints: A key part of good form is protecting your joints, and that means a variety of things depending on the exercise you're doing. In general, some goals to shoot for include:

» Keeping joints slightly bent—In many exercises, you're lifting limbs up, overhead, to the sides, and other directions. What you don't want, generally, is to lock the joints, which can put pressure on them. Many exercises will instruct you to keep a slight bend to avoid that.

» Avoiding undue pressure on the knees—Some exercises, particularly squats, lunges, and other moves that involve bending the knees can cause pain if done incorrectly. In general, you want to put the weight in the heels of your feet and avoid sending the knees too far over the toes. Doing that can place too much weight on the knee joint, which can cause pain and discomfort.

» Keeping your joints in alignment—One other thing to think about is making sure one joint isn't going in the wrong direction. Think of bending forward to pick something up. Imagine if your knee went way out to the side instead of straight forward… you might be in for a knee injury. Paying attention to that during your exercises can keep you safe and injury-free.

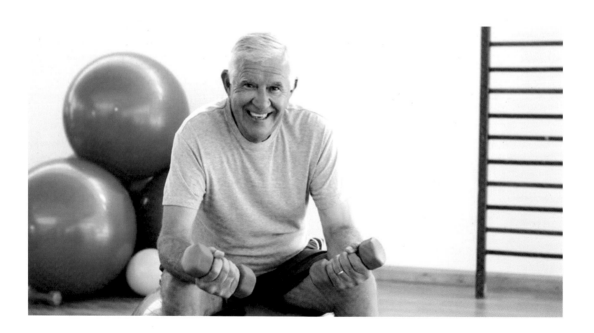

Chapter 6

How the Program Works

This 12-week program is designed to focus attention on the most important aspects of your fitness including strength, endurance, balance, and flexibility. The idea is to work on the things that will give you the most bang for your buck.

It's also designed to gradually progress your fitness in a safe, healthy way so you can perfect the exercises and movements while feeling good in your body.

There are four different types of workouts you'll do over the course of the program. These include:

- ✓ A dynamic warm-up—Exercises designed to get your body ready for more intense exercise and mimic some of the movements you'll be doing during your main workout.
- ✓ Strength training workouts—Your workouts will change over the course of the program, but they include a variety of exercises that hit all the major muscle groups using different types of equipment. Every workout will focus on building whole body strength that translates into everyday activities.
- ✓ Core and balance workouts—These exercises focus close attention on your core, which includes all of the muscles in your abs, pelvis, and back. Balance exercises help you work on mobility and stabilization, which will also translate into real-life activities.
- ✓ Flexibility—Your stretching workout offers simple, easy-to-do exercises that can be done anywhere, anytime to help you relax and improve your range of motion.

THE WARM-UP

The warm-up is one of the most important parts of your workout, a time for you to gradually increase your heart rate, circulation, and bring more oxygen to the muscles.

It also gives you a chance to lubricate your joints and increase your flexibility, all of which will not only make your workout better, but can help protect your body from injury.

Muscles that are warm and relaxed will help you move more easily and with less pain and stiffness, and you'll get a better range of motion once your muscles are warm. Not only does your body do better with a warm-up, it's also a time to get your mind ready for the workout to come.

Your 10-minute warm-up includes eight total body dynamic moves using a very light weight. These exercises are designed to prepare your body for the more intense demands of the strength training workouts.

This warm-up includes a number of exercises that mimic some of the movements you'll be doing in your workout. However, there are other ways you can warm up if you want something different over the course of the program. You can do light cardio exercise such as walking, cycling, or aerobics.

The idea is to do some kind of rhythmic movement so that your muscles are warm, supple, and you feel ready for exercise.

If you're doing a different type of warm-up, make sure it's at least five minutes long and that you work at an easy intensity, gradually increasing how hard you're working so that your body feels warm and ready for exercise.

THE STRENGTH TRAINING WORKOUTS

Your program starts with total body strength training with a variety of movement patterns that not only mimic daily movements, such as squatting and lifting, but also help you build a strong foundation that will support your body in both exercise and daily activities.

This program is set up to ease you into strength training by giving you time to perfect different movement patterns and feel comfortable with challenging your body with different types of resistance.

The workouts include ten or more exercises, some using resistance, such as dumbbells or resistance bands, and others not, that target all the major muscles of the body including the chest, back, shoulders, arms, and legs. Your suggested schedule includes strength training one to two times a week with at least one day of rest in between.

For each exercise, you'll do a number of sets and repetitions that change over the course of the program so that you avoid hitting a plateau. Repetitions refer to how many times you do an exercise while a set is the number of repetitions you do consecutively.

Every two weeks, you'll do a new strength training workout that builds on the previous one with a focus on developing a consistent exercise habit while increasing that all-important lean muscle tissue.

Every two weeks you'll get new workouts as well as a suggested workout schedule so you can plan your week ahead of time.

CORE, BALANCE, AND FLEXIBILITY WORKOUTS

The core and balance workouts are important because they help you strengthen the most important part of your body. Many of our movements originate from the core, and balance is one thing we often struggle with as we get older.

With these exercises, you'll build stronger connective tissue while also working on those important stabilizer muscles in the body. As you do each balance exercise, you'll feel those small muscles, often in your feet and ankles, firing to keep you steady.

All that stability translates into real-life activities like stepping on and off a curb, getting in and out of a car, or going up and down stairs.

The flexibility workout includes stretches for all the major muscle groups and can be done as often as you like, with a minimum of three times a week. This is a great workout to do after your strength training, and much of it is seated so you can relax and focus on feeling good.

THE WORKOUT SCHEDULE

The suggested workout schedules include strength training workouts as well as core and balance training.

On the off days, you can incorporate your own exercise that can include cardio workouts and/or active movement. Some of these activities include:

- ✓ Walking
- ✓ Jogging
- ✓ Swimming
- ✓ Cycling
- ✓ Yard work
- ✓ Household chores
- ✓ Stretching

Off days can be a time for you to rest your muscles if they're sore and you feel tired. Or, off days can offer a time to be active and focus your energy on moving around more than you normally do. This can be as simple as setting an alarm for every hour so you can stand up, move around, and stretch.

Chapter 7

Let's Get Started: The Warm-Up and Flexibility Workout

THE WARM-UP

Do the following dynamic exercises before each strength and core workout. For each exercise, hold a very light weight in both hands. The weight should be between one and three pounds. Complete one set of each exercise. If you feel any pain or discomfort in the joints, ease up on the movement or skip it altogether if you can't do the exercise without pain. You can also do the exercises with no weights until you feel comfortable with the movements.

Note: Each exercise includes pictures as well as instructions. The instructions for each move, as well as the reps and sets, *precede* each exercise.

SQUATS

Hold a light weight at chest level and bend the knees, sending the hips back into a squat. Make sure your knees don't go over your toes but, instead, put your weight in your heels. Stand up and repeat.

1 x 10 reps

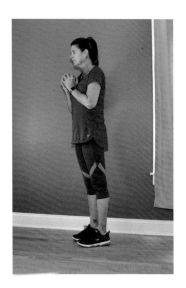
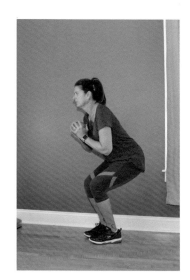

VERTICAL WOODCHOP

Hold a light weight and squat, sending the hips towards the back wall with the weight between the knees. Stand and swing the weight up and overhead. Lower and repeat.

    1 x 10 reps

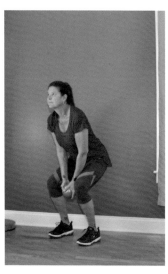
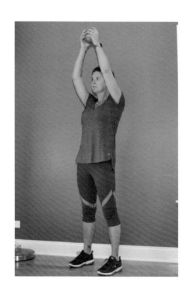

REVERSE LUNGE

Holding a light weight with the feet together, step back with the right foot about 2 to 3 feet, bend the knees, and lower into a lunge. Make sure you go straight down, taking the right knee towards the floor, keeping the front knee behind the toes. Step back to start and repeat, alternating sides.

   1 x 16 reps

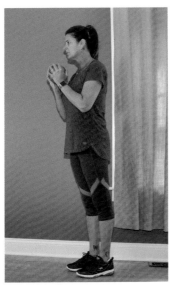 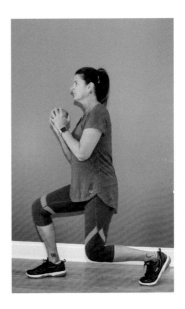

SIDE LUNGE

Holding a light weight at the chest step out to the right, keeping the left leg straight. Bend the right knee, sending the hips back, and lower into a side lunge. Step back to start and alternate sides.

   1 x 16 reps

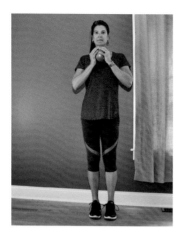 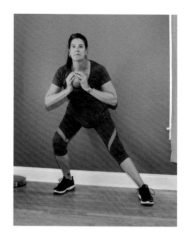

REVERSE LUNGE WITH ROTATION

Hold a light weight at torso level and step back into a reverse lunge with the right foot. As you bend the knees into a lunge, gently rotate the torso to the right. Step back and take the left foot back into a reverse lunge, gently rotating the torso to the left. Step back to start and repeat, alternating sides.

1 x 16 reps

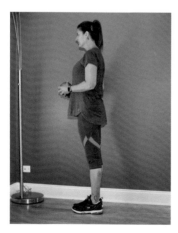 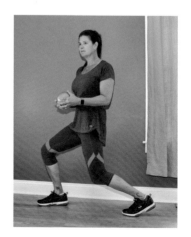

SQUAT WITH A ROTATING PRESS

Holding a light weight in the left hand, bend the knees, sending the hips back into a squat. As you stand, rotate to the right while pressing the weight up overhead. Switch hands, lower into a squat, and press up, rotating to the left and pressing the weight up with the right hand. Repeat all reps on that side before switching sides.

   1 x 10 reps

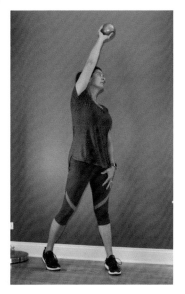 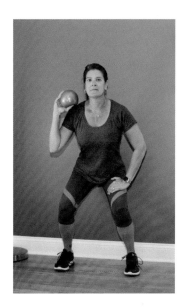

NARROW SQUAT WITH ALTERNATING ROWS

Hold a light weight in both hands while standing with the feet close together. Bend the knees into a squat and tip forward from the hips a bit, keeping the back straight with the weight straight out in front of you. Holding the squat, pull the weight back in a rowing motion with the right hand, squeezing the back. Return back to start and repeat, alternating sides.

   1 x 16 reps

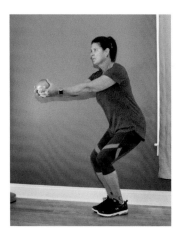 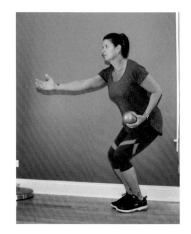

SPLIT STANCE WITH CROSS-BODY ROTATION

Stand in a staggered stance with the left foot back and the right knee slightly bent. Keep your feet wide for better balance and hold a light weight in the left hand. Keeping the left arm straight, take the weight straight back behind you, turning to look at the weight. Return to start and repeat, alternating sides. If this throws you off balance, look forward instead of back.

   1 x 10 reps

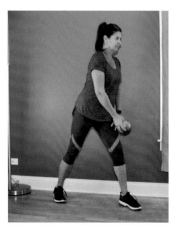 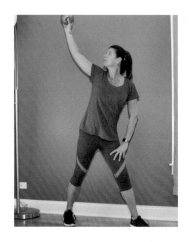

FLEXIBILITY WORKOUT

This workout can be done two to three times a week, either after a workout or on its own for flexibility and relaxation. This gentle workout can also be done on a daily basis and is a great way to stay active when you're doing something more sedentary, such as watching TV.

EQUIPMENT NEEDED
A sturdy chair.

SEATED TORSO STRETCH
Sit tall and lace the fingers together, taking the arms straight up towards the ceiling and stretching through the torso. Without lifting the hips, stretch the arms up and over to the right, stretching the left side of the torso. Hold for 15 to 30 seconds and repeat on the other side.

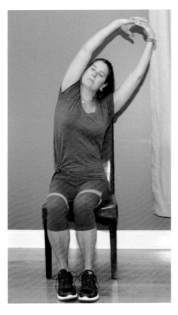 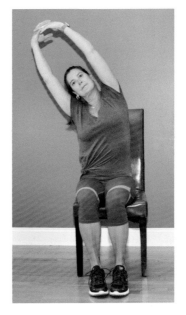

SEATED TRICEPS STRETCH

Sit tall and reach both arms up, palms facing in. Bend the right elbow, taking the hand behind the head and gently pull on the elbow with the left hand, feeling a stretch in the back of the arm. Hold for 15 to 30 seconds and repeat on the other side.

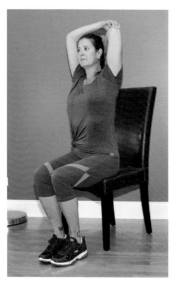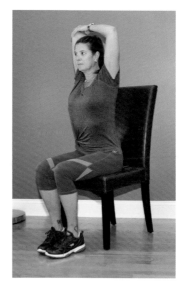

BICEPS STRETCH

Sit tall and take the arms straight out to the sides with the thumbs pointing up. Rotate the hands so the thumbs face down and gently press your arms towards the back of the room, stretching the arms. Hold for 15 to 30 seconds.

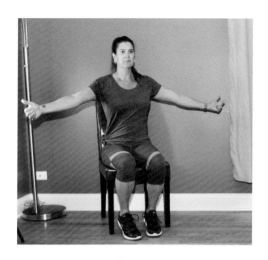 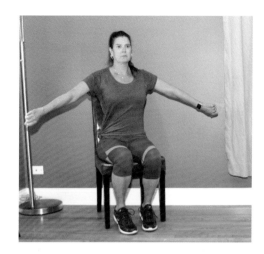

UPPER BACK STRETCH

In a seated position, lace the fingers together and stretch up overhead. Then round the back while contracting the abs and stretch the arms towards the front of the room, stretching the upper back. Hold for 15 to 30 seconds.

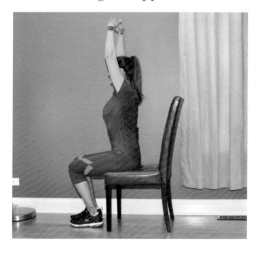 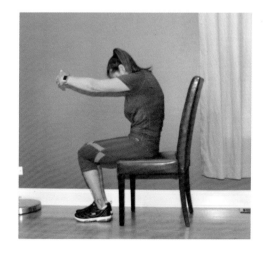

SEATED HIP STRETCH

Sit tall and cross the right ankle over the left knee. Gently press forward, keeping the back straight, and feel a stretch in the right hip. You can also gently press down on the right knee for a deeper stretch. Hold for 15 to 30 seconds and switch sides.

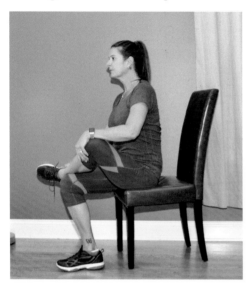 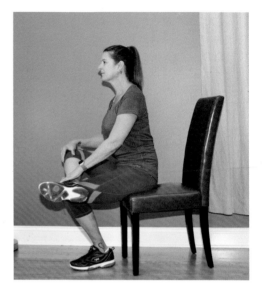

SEATED HAMSTRING STRETCH

Sit tall and take the right leg straight out and rest on the heel, foot flexed. With the back flat, gently lean forward until you feel a stretch in the back of the right leg. Hold for 15 to 30 seconds and repeat on the other side.

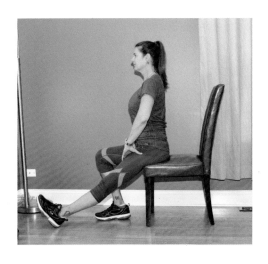
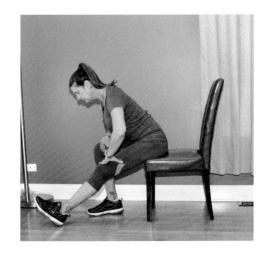

STANDING HIP FLEXOR STRETCH

Stand behind a chair and hold on for balance. Take the right foot back behind you and bend both knees into a half lunge. Squeeze the right glute, pressing forward and feeling a stretch in the front of the right hip. Hold for 15 to 30 seconds and repeat on the other side.

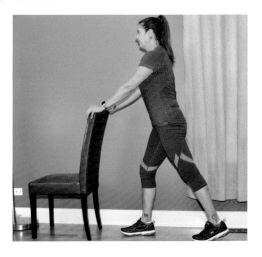
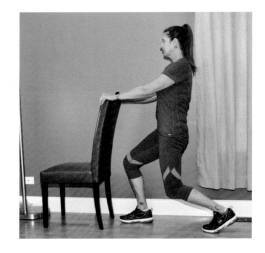

STANDING CAT-COW

From a standing position, bend the knees and place the hands on the thighs. Pressing gently on the thighs, round the back, reaching the upper back towards the ceiling, keeping the abs in. Release the back and return to a flat back. Smoothly move back and forth between the motions for 15 reps.

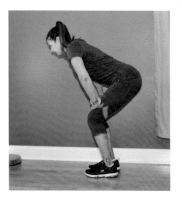 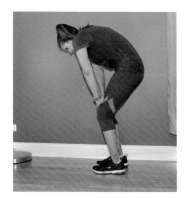

CALF STRETCH

Stand next to a wall or chair for balance and take the right leg back behind you, leg straight. Press the right heel down to the floor and gently press forward until you feel a stretch in the back of the right calf. Hold for 15 to 30 seconds and switch sides.

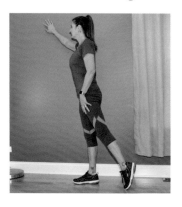 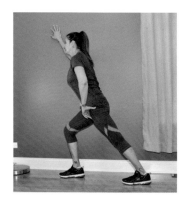

Chapter 8
Total Body Strength: Weeks 1 and 2

This first workout eases you into your journey of getting strong and fit. Begin with the warm-up workout, or your own warm-up, and then complete each exercise with the suggested reps and sets. During Week 1, do one set of each exercise. During Week 2, do two sets of each exercise, resting for 10 to 30 seconds in between each set.

Be sure to skip any exercise that causes pain.

EQUIPMENT NEEDED
For women, light: 2 to 5 lbs, medium: 5 to 8 lbs, heavy: 8 to 10 lbs
For men, light: 5 to 8 lbs, medium: 8 to 10 lbs, heavy: 10 to 12 lbs
Gliding discs or other sliding equipment (e.g., towels or paper plates)
A sturdy, unmoving chair

SUGGESTED WORKOUT SCHEDULE
Day 1: Total Body Strength 1/Flexibility
Day 2: Rest or active movement
Day 3: Total Body Strength 1/Flexibility
Day 4: Rest or active movement
Day 5: Rest or active movement
Day 6: Core and Balance Workout 1
Day 7: Flexibility

SIT AND STANDS

Stand in front of a sturdy chair and bend the knees, sitting lightly on the edge of the chair. Press into the heels to stand all the way up while trying not to use your hands.

1 x 16 reps

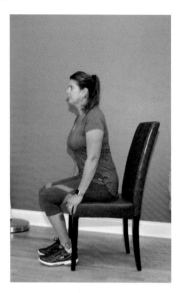 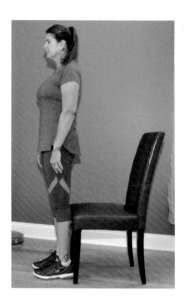

ASSISTED LUNGES

Stand next to a wall or chair for balance and stand in a split stance, the left leg back and the right leg forward about three feet apart. Bend the knees and lower the back knee towards the floor, keeping the front knee behind the toe. Keep the torso straight and abs in as you push back to start. Repeat on the same side before switching legs.

1 x 12 reps

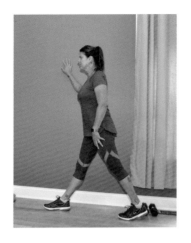 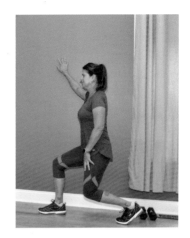

SEATED DOUBLE ARM ROWS

Hold weights in each hand as you sit on the edge of a sturdy chair. Lean forward, keeping the back straight and the abs in, hanging the weights down on either side of the legs. Bend the elbows and row them up to torso level, squeezing the back muscles. Lower and repeat. Suggested weights: medium.

1 x 12 reps

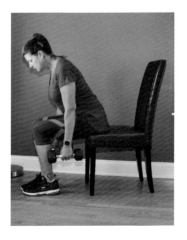 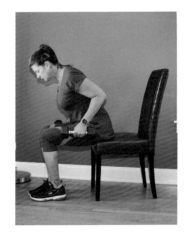

LATERAL RAISE

Stand tall with good posture and hold weights in both hands with the palms facing out right next to the hips. Lift the arms straight up to the sides just to shoulder level. Lower and repeat. Suggested weights: light.

   1 x 12 reps

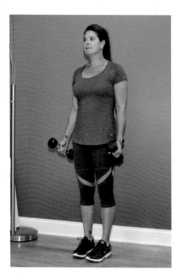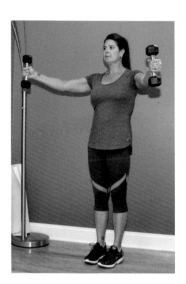

BICEPS CURL

Stand tall with good posture and hold weights in both hands with the palms facing out just in front of the thighs. Bend the elbows and curl the weights up towards the shoulders, squeezing the biceps. Lower and repeat. Suggested weights: medium.

   1 x 12 reps

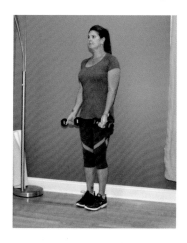 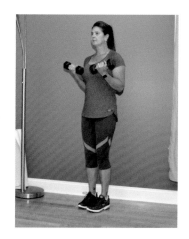

SEATED TRICEPS EXTENSIONS

Sit tall in a sturdy chair and hold one weight in both hands. Take the weight straight up overhead and keep the core engaged. Bend the elbows, lowering the weight behind your head until the elbows are at about 90-degree angles. Squeeze the back of the arms to lift the weight back up and repeat. Suggested weight: heavy.

1 x 12 reps

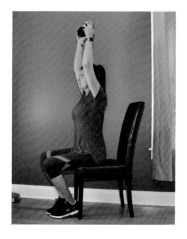 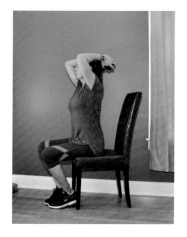

WALL PUSH-UPS

Stand about 2 feet from a wall with your arms straight out in front of you, palms on the wall. Your hands should be shoulder-width apart and at shoulder height. Bend the elbows and lean your body towards the wall until your nose almost touches it. Keep your back straight and abs in. Push back to start and repeat. You can adjust the difficulty by standing closer (easier) or further away (harder).

   1 x 12 reps

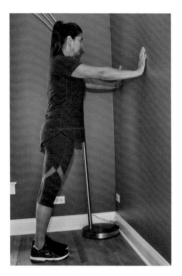 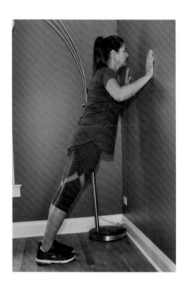

SEATED CALF RAISES

Sit tall at the edge of a chair and place the palms on the thighs. Press down into the thighs as you lift up onto the toes, squeezing the calves. Lower and repeat.

   1 x 12 reps

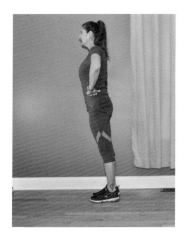 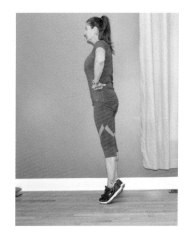

SEATED LEG EXTENSIONS

Sit tall at the edge of a chair and cross the arms over the chest (more difficult) or keep them on either side of the chair. Squeeze the right thigh as you extend the right leg straight, keeping the left foot on the ground. Lower and repeat all reps on one side before switching sides.

   1 x 12 reps

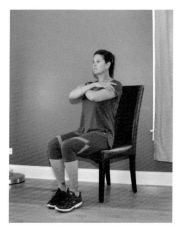 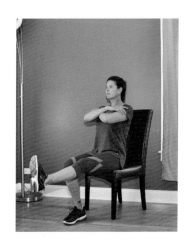

CHAIR HEEL SLIDES

Sit tall on a chair with gliding devices under each heel, feet flexed. Press the right heel into the gliding device and slide the leg out. Continue to press into the gliding device to slide the right heel back in. Repeat, alternating sides.

   1 x 16 reps

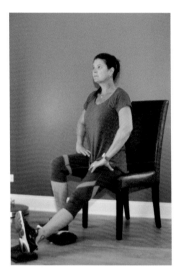 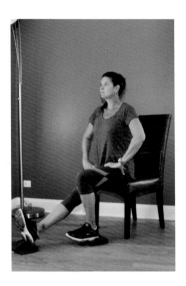

CORE AND BALANCE WORKOUT 1

Begin with the warm-up workout or your own light warm-up. Complete each exercise as shown for the suggested time and/or reps, skipping any moves that cause pain or discomfort.

EQUIPMENT NEEDED

A sturdy, unmoving chair
One medium weight

KNEE LIFT AND HOLD

Stand behind a chair and hold on with both hands for balance. Lift the right knee up and hold for as long as you can, up to 30 seconds. Lower and repeat on the other side.

1 x 3 reps on each side

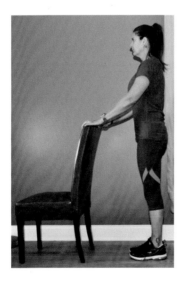
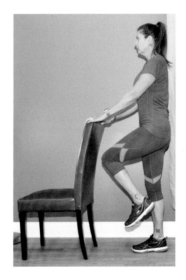

REAR LEG LIFT

Stand behind a chair and hold on with one hand for balance. Keeping the core engaged and the back straight, lift the right leg straight behind you, keeping the leg straight and squeezing the glutes. Lower and repeat on the same side before switching legs.

1 x 15 reps

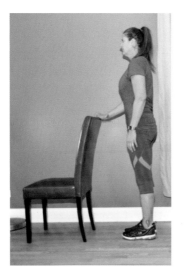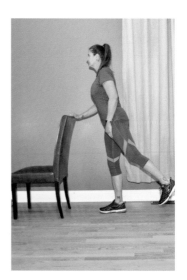

CLOCK REACH

Hold on to a chair with your left hand and lift your right knee. Hold the knee up as you reach forward with the right hand towards what would be 12 on a clock. Next point your arm to 3 and, finally, point behind you at 6. Bring your arm back to number 3, then to 12, looking straight the entire time.

1 x 2 reps on each side

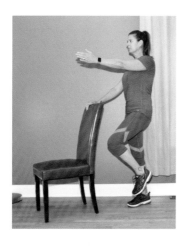 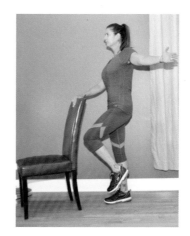

SAME SIDE KNEE/ARM LIFT

Stand in front of a chair and hold on with the right hand for balance. Raise your left hand over your head and slowly raise the left foot off the floor. Hold for 10 seconds and repeat, alternating sides.

  1 x 3 reps on each side

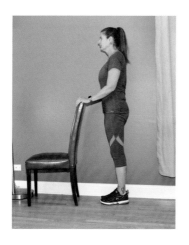 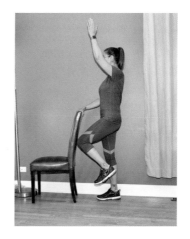

SIDE LEG LIFT WITH CHAIR

Stand and hold on to a chair for balance. Shift the weight to the left foot as you lift the right leg straight out to the side as high as you can without moving or tilting the torso. Lower and repeat all reps before switching sides.

   1 x 16 reps

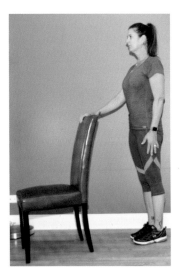 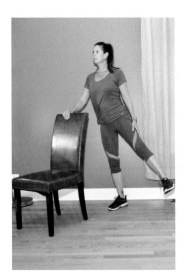

SEATED SIDE BENDS

Sit tall at the edge of a chair and lace the hands behind the head, elbows out. Keeping the hips and knees facing forward, lean to the right as far as you can, squeezing the right side of the waist. Return to start and repeat, alternating sides.

   1 x 16 reps

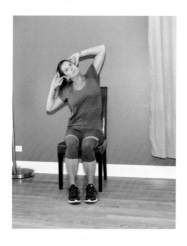 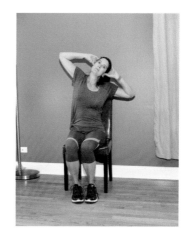

SEATED ROTATIONS

Sit tall and hold a medium weight in both hands at chest level, elbows parallel to the floor. Keeping the hips and knees facing forward, squeeze the weight and rotate to the right as far as you can. Return to the center and repeat, alternating sides.

  1 x 16 reps

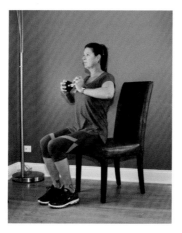 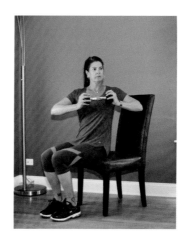

SEATED CROSSOVER CRUNCHES

Sit tall and lace the hands behind the head, elbows out. Lift the right knee and rotate the opposite shoulder across the body, squeezing the right side of the waist. Lower and repeat, alternating sides. Keep the elbows out the entire time instead of bending them forward.

　1 x 16 reps

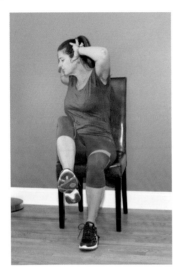 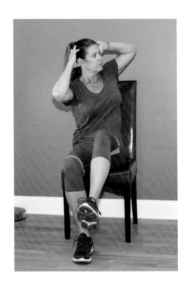

CHAIR PRESS-UPS

Sit tall and place the hands on either side of the hips. Press into the chair and lift the hips a few inches off the chair, bracing the core. Lower and repeat.

　1 x 12 reps

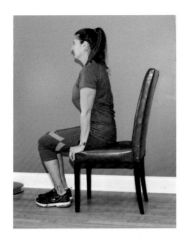 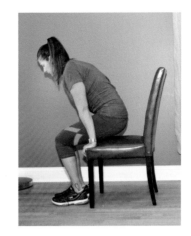

CHAIR KNEE LIFTS

Sit tall and grip either side of the chair. Keeping the back straight, gently lift the feet off the ground, keeping the knees bent and squeezing the lower abs. Lower and repeat.

1 x 12 reps

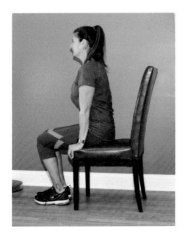 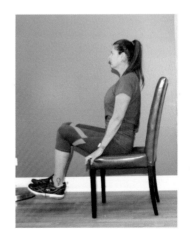

Chapter 9
Total Body Strength 2:
Weeks 3 and 4

This week you'll have new exercises to take you to the next level in building strength and fitness. The exercises will be familiar, but with a twist that helps you build on everything you've worked on during the first two weeks.

Begin with your warm-up and then complete each exercise as shown for the suggested reps and sets. As with the previous workout, do one set of each exercise during Week 3 and, during Week 4, do two sets with a 10- to 30-second rest between each set.

As before, skip any exercise that causes pain.

EQUIPMENT NEEDED

Light, medium, and heavy weights

A sturdy, unmoving chair

A mat

SUGGESTED WORKOUT SCHEDULE

Day 1: Total Body Strength 2/Flexibility

Day 2: Rest or active movement

Day 3: Total Body Strength 2/Flexibility

Day 4: Rest or active movement

Day 5: Rest or active movement

Day 6: Core and Balance Workout 1

Day 7: Flexibility

HOVER SIT AND STAND

Stand in front of a sturdy chair and hold a weight in both hands at chest level. Bend the knees and squat as though you're going to sit down, but stop just before you sit all the way down. Press into the heels to stand and repeat. Suggested weights: heavy.

1 x 12 reps

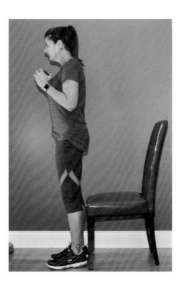 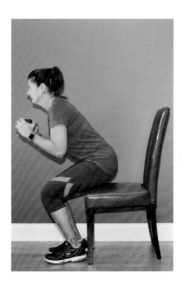

REVERSE LUNGES

Holding weights in each hand, step back with the right foot about 2 to 3 feet and bend the knees and lower into a lunge. Make sure you go straight down, taking the right knee towards the floor, keeping the front knee behind the toes. Step back to start and repeat on the same side before switching sides. Suggested weights: light.

1 x 12 reps

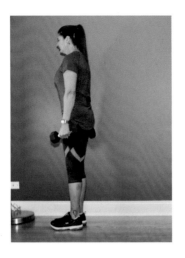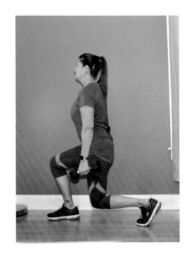

GOOD MORNINGS

Stand tall and hold a weight in both hands behind the head. Keeping the back straight and with a slight bend in the knees, tip from the hips and lean forward (back flat) until you're parallel to the floor or you feel a stretch in the back of your thighs. Return to start and repeat. Suggested weight: light.

   1 x 12 reps

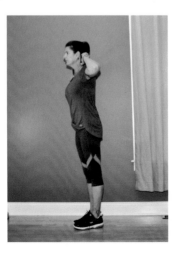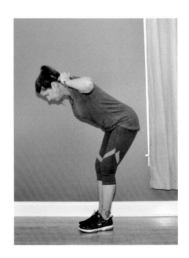

SINGLE ARM DUMBBELL ROW

Stand behind a chair and hold on with the right hand for balance. Hold a weight in the left hand and tip from the hips with the back flat until the torso is at about a 45-degree angle, weight hanging down. Bend the elbow and pull the weight up, bringing the elbow to the torso squeezing the back. Lower and and repeat for all reps before switching sides. Suggested weight: heavy.

    1 x 12 reps

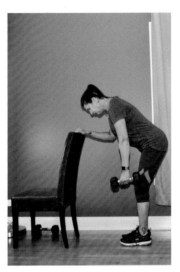 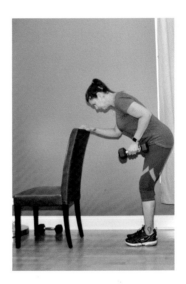

LATERAL RAISE

Stand tall with good posture and hold weights in both hands with the palms facing out right next to the hips. Lift the arms straight up to the sides just to shoulder level. Lower and repeat. Suggested weights: light to medium.

    1 x 12 reps

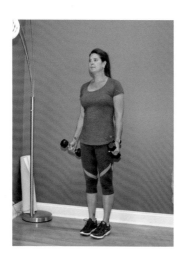 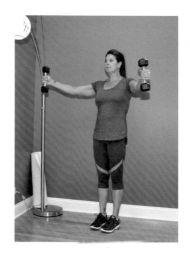

OVERHEAD PRESS

Stand with feet hip-width apart and hold weights with the elbows bent and in line with the shoulders like a goal post. Keeping the core engaged, press the weights up overhead. Return to start and repeat. Suggested weights: light.

   1 x 12 reps

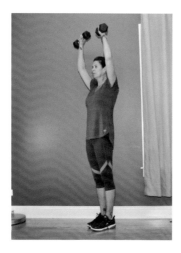 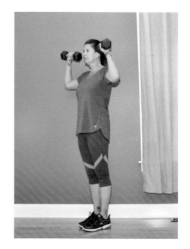

HAMMER CURLS

Stand with feet hip-width apart and hold weights in both hands next to the thighs, palms facing in. Bend the elbows and curl the weights up to shoulder level, keeping the palms facing in. Lower and repeat. Suggested weights: medium.

   1 x 12 reps

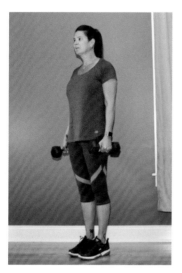
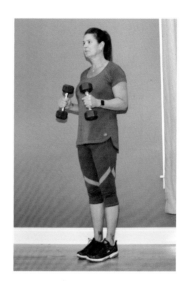

STANDING TRICEPS EXTENSIONS

Holding one weight in both hands, place the feet about hip-width apart and take the weight straight up. Bend the elbows, taking the weight behind your head until your elbows are at 90-degree angles. Squeeze the back of the arms to lift the weight back up and repeat. Suggested weight: medium to heavy.

   1 x 12 reps

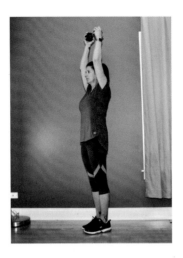 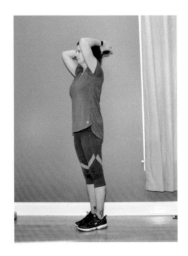

STRAIGHT LEG RAISES

Stand next to a wall or chair for balance. Flex the right foot and lift the right leg straight up as far as you can without tilting the torso back. Lower and repeat for all reps before switching sides.

   1 x 12 reps

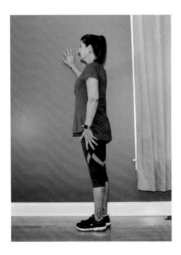 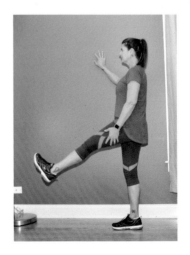

MODIFIED FLOOR PUSH-UPS

Using your mat, get on all fours with the hands about shoulder-width apart. Bend the elbows and keep the back straight as you bring your nose towards the mat. Press back up and repeat. To make it harder, walk the hands forward to put more weight on the upper body.

   1 x 12 reps

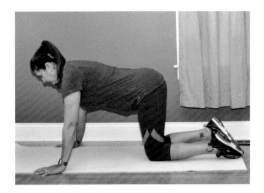 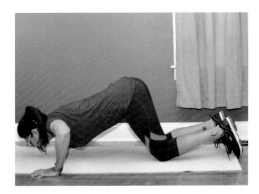

CHEST PRESSES

Lie down with the knees bent and hold weights in both hands directly over the chest. Bend the elbows and lower them towards the floor, just briefly touching at the bottom. The arms should look like goal posts. Press the weight back up and repeat. Suggested weights: light to medium.

   1 x 12 reps

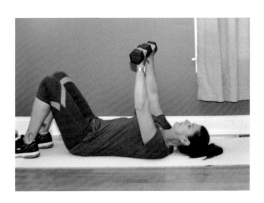 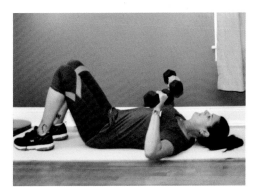

Chapter 10
Total Body Strength 3: Weeks 5 and 6

Your workouts continue progress with new and challenging exercises this week. Begin with your warm up and then perform each exercise as shown. During Week 5, do one set of each exercise. During Week 6, do two sets of each exercise with 10 to 30 seconds of rest in between sets.

Be sure to skip any exercise that causes pain.

EQUIPMENT NEEDED

Light, medium, and heavy weights
A sturdy, unmoving chair
A light to medium tension resistance band
A mat

SUGGESTED WORKOUT SCHEDULE

Day 1: Total Body Strength 3/Flexibility
Day 2: Rest or active movement
Day 3: Total Body Strength 3/Flexibility
Day 4: Rest or active movement
Day 5: Rest or active movement
Day 6: Core and Balance Workout 2
Day 7: Flexibility

SQUATS WITH WEIGHTS

Stand with feet about hip-width apart and hold weights in both hands at your sides. Bend the knees and send the hips back, squatting as low as you can. Press up and repeat. Suggested weights: medium to heavy.

   1 x 12 reps

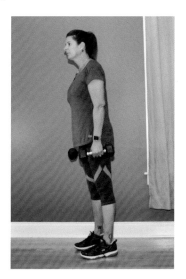 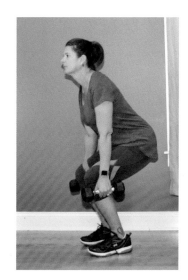

FORWARD LUNGES

Stand with feet together and hold weights in both hands. Step forward with the right foot about two to three feet in front of you. Bend the knees and bring the back knee straight down towards the floor. Press into the heel to return to start and repeat for all reps before switching sides. Suggested weights: light to medium.

   1 x 12 reps

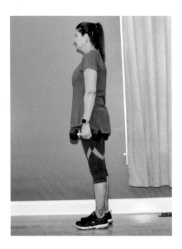
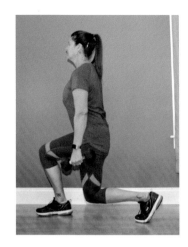

DEADLIFTS

Stand with the feet about hip-width apart and hold weights in front of the thighs. With the knees slightly bent, tip from the hips, keeping the back straight and the abs in while taking the weight towards the floor. Don't round at the shoulders, but keep the back flat and keep the weights close to the body like you're shaving your legs. Squeeze the butt to lift up and repeat. Suggested weights: Heavy.

1 x 12 reps

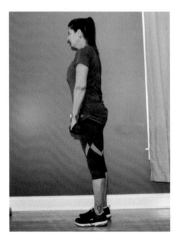
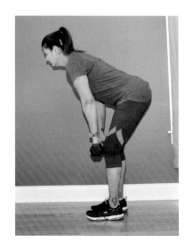

KNEE LIFTS WITH BANDS

Take a light to medium resistance band and tie it around your ankles with about three inches between your ankles. You may need to adjust the length to increase or decrease the tension in the band. Holding on to a chair for balance, lift the right knee up as high as you can, feeling it in the front of the thigh. Lower and repeat for all reps before switching sides.

1 x 12 reps

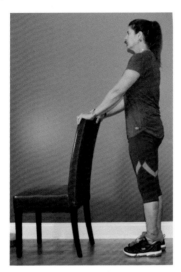 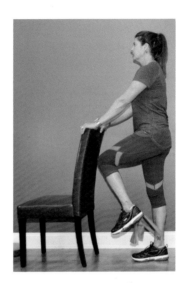

HAMSTRING CURLS WITH BANDS

Take a light to medium resistance band and tie it around your ankles and position the band so that it's under the right foot and around the left ankle. Keeping the foot flexed and holding on to a chair for balance, lift the heel towards the glutes, squeezing the back of the thigh. Lower and repeat for all reps before switching sides.

1 x 12 reps

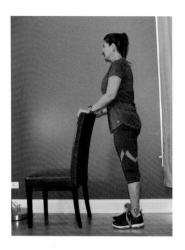 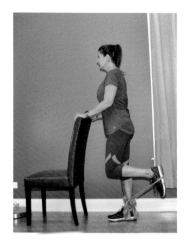

REAR FLIES WITH BANDS

Stand holding a light to medium resistance band in both hands a few inches apart. You may need to adjust your hand position to make this exercise easier or harder. Taking the arms straight out in front of you, open the hands and squeeze the shoulder blades together as you take the arms straight back, stopping at torso level. Return to start and repeat.

1 x 12 reps

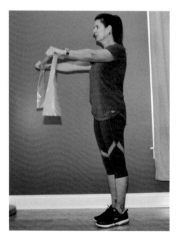 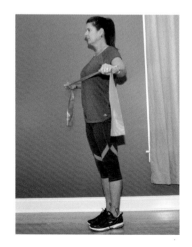

ONE ARM DUMBBELL ROW

Stand with the right leg back in a staggered stance, right leg straight and the left leg bent. Hold a weight in the left hand and rest the right hand on the front thigh to support the lower back. Tip forward, back straight and the weight hanging down. Bend the elbows and pull the weight up, bringing the elbow to torso level and squeezing the back. Lower and repeat for all reps before switching sides. Suggested weights: heavy.

1 x 12 reps

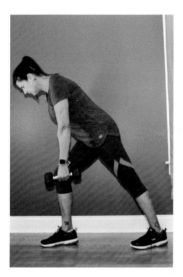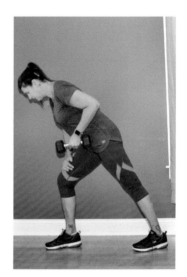

OVERHEAD PRESS

Stand with feet hip-width apart and hold weights with the elbows bent and in line with the shoulders like a goal post. Keeping the core engaged, press the weights up overhead. Return to start and repeat. Suggested weights: light.

1 x 12 reps

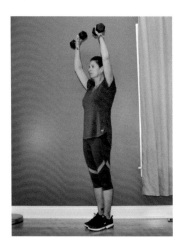 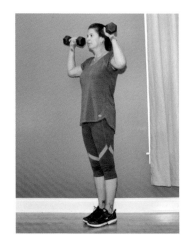

FRONT RAISE

Stand with feet hip-width apart and hold weights directly in front of the thighs, palms facing the thighs. Keeping the core engaged, lift the weights straight up in front of you to shoulder level. Lower and repeat. Suggested weights: light.

  1 x 12 reps

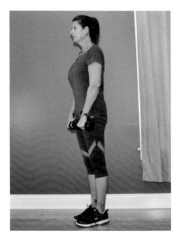 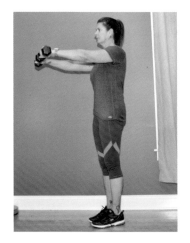

ROTATING BICEPS CURLS

Stand with feet hip-width apart and hold weights at your sides with the palms facing in. Bend the elbows to curl the weights up towards the shoulders, rotating the hands so that they're facing the shoulders at the top of the movement. Lower and repeat. Suggested weights: medium to heavy.

   1 x 12 reps

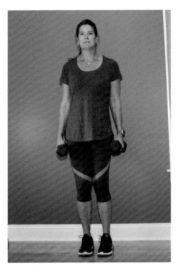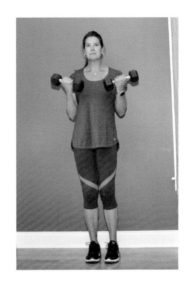

KICKBACKS

Stand with feet hip-width apart and hold weights in each hand. Tip from the hips, abs engaged and the back flat, tilting forward to about 45 degrees. Pull the elbows up to torso level and, holding that position, extend the arms, taking the weights behind you and squeezing the back of the arms. Lower the weights and repeat. Suggested weights: light to medium.

   1 x 12 reps

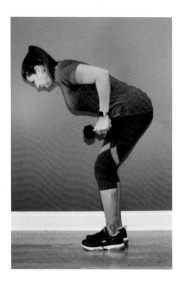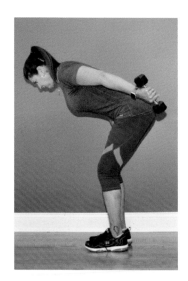

MODIFIED FLOOR PUSH-UPS

Using your mat, get on all fours with the hands about shoulder-width apart. Bend the elbows and keep the back straight as you bring your nose towards the mat. Press back up and repeat. To make it harder, walk the hands forward to put more weight on the upper body.

1 x 12 reps

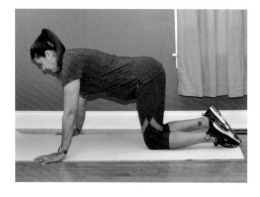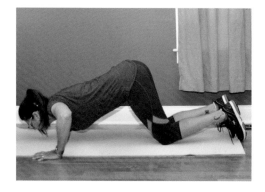

CHEST PRESSES

Lie down with the knees bent and hold weights in both hands directly over the chest. Bend the elbows and lower them towards the floor, just briefly touching at the bottom. The arms should look like goal posts. Press the weight back up and repeat. Suggested weights: medium.

   1 x 12 reps

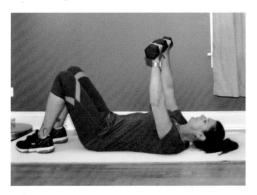 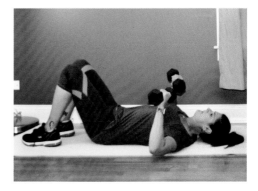

CORE AND BALANCE WORKOUT 2

Your next core and balance workout includes a variety of new standing and floor exercises. Complete each exercise as shown for the time and/or reps shown, skipping any moves that cause pain or discomfort.

EQUIPMENT NEEDED

A sturdy chair
A mat

LEG LIFT

Stand tall with the hands on the hips. Shift the weight to your left leg as you slowly lift the right leg out to the side, foot flexed. Lift it as high as you can without tilting to the other side. Lower and repeat for all reps before switching sides.

   1 x 16 reps

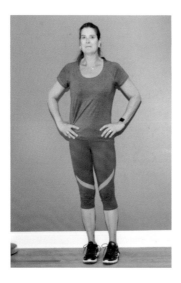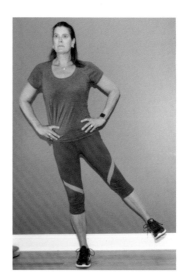

HEEL TO TOE WALK

Begin at one end of the room and step forward with the right foot. Bring the left foot in front of the right, taking the left heel in front of the right foot. Now step the right foot forward, bringing the right heel in front of the left foot. You may need to hold on to a wall for balance at first. Continue across the room then turn around and come back, completing three laps.

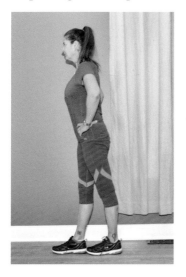 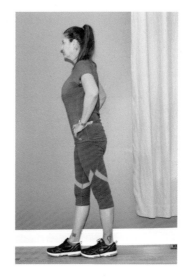

ROCK THE BOAT

Stand with the feet wide, hands on the hips. Shift your weight to the left leg and lift the right knee up, taking the foot a few inches off the ground. Step back down and shift to the right, lifting the left leg up. Continue going from side to side.

1 x 16 reps

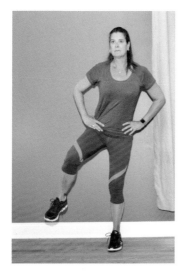 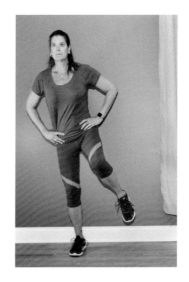

CALF RAISE

Stand next to a wall for balance if needed and lift the heels as high as you can, squeezing the calves. Lower and repeat.

    1 x 16 reps

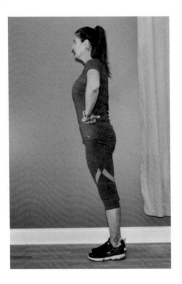 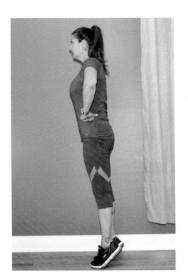

OVER THE SHOULDER WALK

Starting at one end of the room, slowly take a step forward with one foot. At the same time, turn your head and look over your opposite shoulder. Keep looking in that direction as you slowly walk across the room. On the way back, look over the other shoulder as you walk. Repeat for 3 laps.

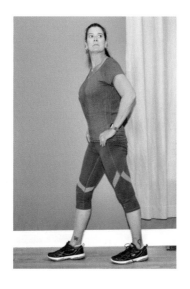
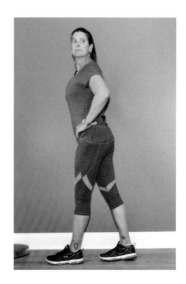

FLOOR CORE LEAN AND LIFT

Sit on your mat with the knees bent and hold on to the back of the thighs for support if needed. Keeping the hands on the knees, round back as far as you can, squeezing the core. Lift back up and repeat. To make it more challenging, take the hands off the knees and reach forward.

   1 x 16 reps

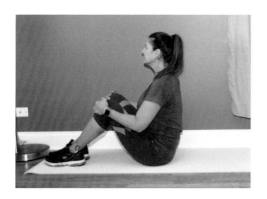
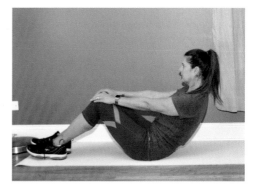

CRUNCH AND REACH

Lie down on your mat with the knees bent. Take your left hand behind your head for support, gently cradling the head (try not to pull on the neck). Take the right hand straight up, contract the abs, and lift the shoulders off the floor as you reach towards the wall with the right hand. Lower and repeat for all reps before switching sides.

1 x 12 reps

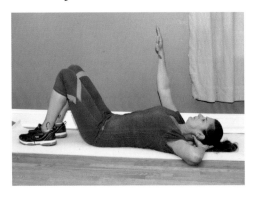 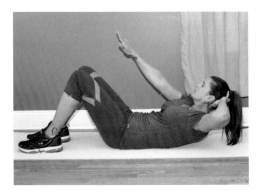

CROSSOVER CRUNCHES

Lying on your mat with the knees bent, cross the left ankle over the right knee. Take the right hand behind the head for support and squeeze the abs to lift the shoulder blades off the floor. Rotate the torso, bringing the right shoulder towards the left hip and squeezing the left side of the waist. Lower and repeat for all reps before switching sides.

1 x 12 reps

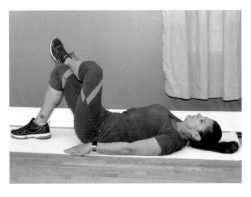 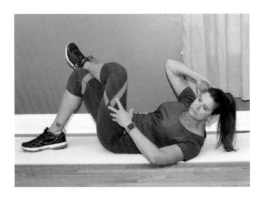

BRIDGES

Lie down on your mat with the knees bent and the hands at your sides. Press into your heels to lift the hips up until your body is in a straight line from the knees to the hips. Slowly lower and repeat.

   1 x 16 reps

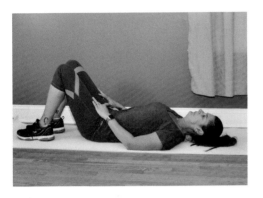 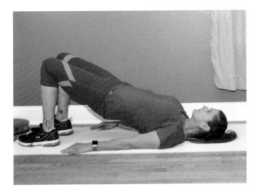

BIRD DOG

Get on the hands and knees, with the hands directly under the shoulders and the knees directly under the hips. Slowly lift the left arm straight up and then lift your right leg straight out so that each is pointed in the opposite direction. Lower and repeat, alternating sides.

   1 x 16 reps

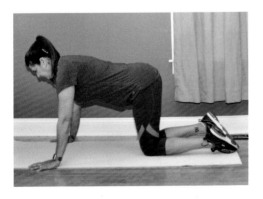 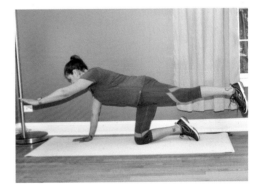

Chapter 11

Split Strength Training: Weeks 7 and 8

Now that you're further into the program, we're going to change things up in the next two weeks by splitting the routine so that you're doing an upper body workout and a lower body workout, along with your core and balance workout.

This allows you to do shorter workouts while focusing more attention on your individual muscle groups, building more strength, muscle, and functionality.

Begin with your warm-up, and then do each move for the suggested reps and sets. Do one set during Week 7, and two sets during Week 8, skipping any exercise that causes any discomfort or pain.

EQUIPMENT NEEDED

Light, medium, and heavy weights
Light to medium tension resistance band
A sturdy, unmoving chair
A mat

SUGGESTED WORKOUT SCHEDULE

Day 1: Upper Body Strength 1/Flexibility
Day 2: Rest or active movement
Day 3: Lower Body Strength 1/Flexibility
Day 4: Rest or active movement
Day 5: Rest or active movement
Day 6: Core and Balance Workout 2
Day 7: Flexibility

UPPER BODY WORKOUT 1

BAND ROWS

Loop the band under the feet and grab on to both handles. Tip from the hips, back flat and abs in until you're almost parallel to the floor. Bend the elbows, pulling them up to torso level while squeezing either side of the back. If you need more tension, grab the band closer to the feet or loop the bands around your hands.

   1 x 12 reps

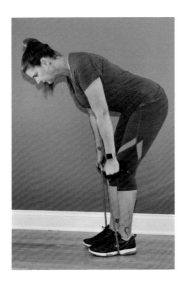 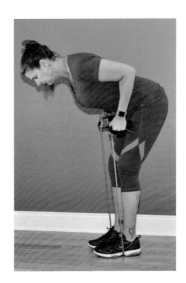

DOUBLE ARM DUMBBELL ROWS

Holding weights in both hands, tip from the hips with a flat back, abs in. Bend the elbows, pulling the weights up in a rowing motion. Lower and repeat. Suggested weights: heavy.

   1 x 12 reps

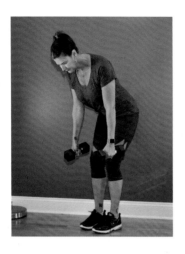
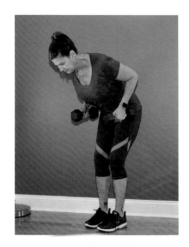

BENT OVER REVERSE FLIES

Sit on the edge of a chair and hold weights as you tip forward, keeping the back flat and the abs in. Squeeze the shoulder blades as you lift the arms straight out to the sides, elbows slightly bent and feeling it in the upper back and shoulders. Lower and repeat. Suggested weights: light.

  1 x 12 reps

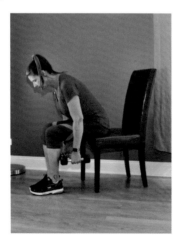
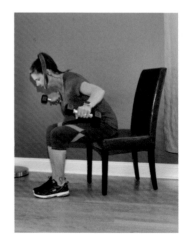

ONE ARM OVERHEAD PRESS

Sit tall and hold one weight in the right hand with the elbow bent, weight on the same level as the ear. Brace the abs and press the weight overhead. Lower and repeat for all reps before switching sides. Suggested weight: medium to heavy.

   1 x 12 reps

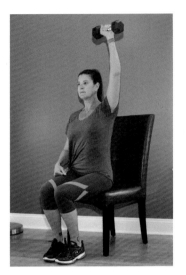 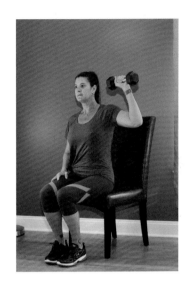

BAND EXTERNAL ROTATIONS

Sit or stand and hold a resistance band in both hands in front of the torso, palms facing up. Keeping the shoulders down, squeeze the shoulder blades and open the hands out to the sides. Keep the elbows in the same position at the torso. Return to start and repeat. Take your hands closer if you need more of a challenge.

   1 x 12 reps

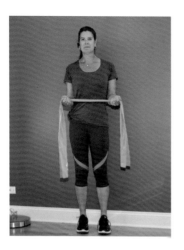 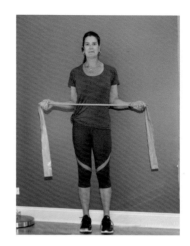

BAND BICEPS CURLS

Loop a resistance band under one foot or both feet (more challenging). Hold the handles in each hand and bend the elbows, curling the weight up towards the shoulders. Slowly lower and repeat.

  1 x 12 reps

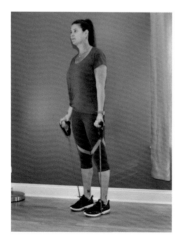 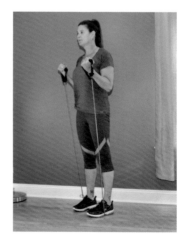

CONCENTRATION CURLS

Sit on a chair and hold one weight in the right hand. Bend forward, supporting your body with the left hand and hang the weight down on the inside of the right thigh. Using your thigh as leverage, curl the weight up towards the shoulder. Slowly lower and repeat for all reps before switching sides. Suggested weight: heavy.

   1 x 12 reps

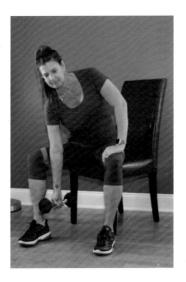 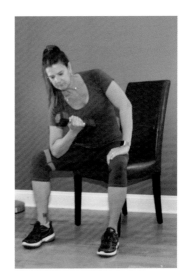

BAND TRICEPS EXTENSIONS

Sit or stand and hold a resistance band in both hands a few inches apart. Bring the hands up to chest level, elbows out and parallel to the ground. Slowly straighten the right arm out, squeezing the back of the arms. Return to start and repeat for all reps before switching sides.

   1 x 12 reps

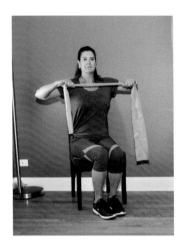 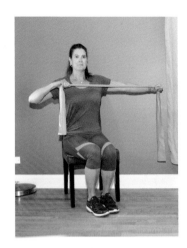

ONE-ARM TRICEPS EXTENSIONS

Stand and hold a weight in the right hand straight up overhead. Place the left hand on the back of the right arm for support. Bend the right elbow, taking the weight behind the head. Squeeze the back of the arm to take the weight straight up again. Repeat for all reps before switching sides. Suggested weight: light to medium.

  1 x 12 reps

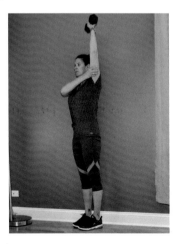 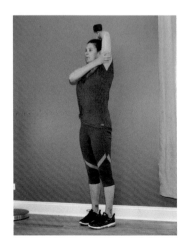

PUSH-UPS

Get on all fours and slowly walk the hands forward until your back is flat and in a straight line, hands shoulder-width apart. Bend the elbows and keep the back straight as you bring your nose towards the mat. Press back up and repeat. If this is challenging, walk the hands back a bit.

1 x 12 reps

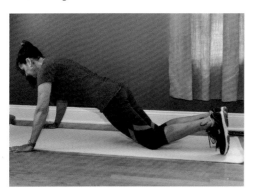 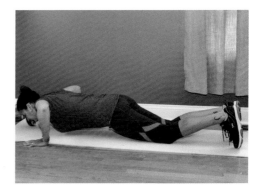

CHEST FLIES

Lie on a mat with the knees bent, and hold weights straight up over the chest with the palms facing in. Keeping a slight bend in the elbows, open the arms out to the sides, gently lowering your arms until they just touch the mat. Return to start and repeat. Suggested weights: light to medium.

1 x 12 reps

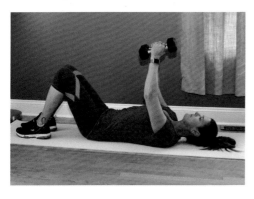 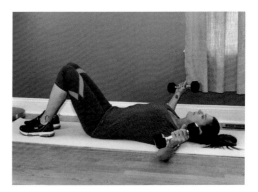

LOWER BODY WORKOUT 1

SQUATS WITH WEIGHTS

Stand with feet about hip-width apart and hold weights in both hands at your sides. Bend the knees and send the hips back, squatting as low as you can. Press up and repeat. Suggested weights: medium to heavy.

   1 x 12 reps

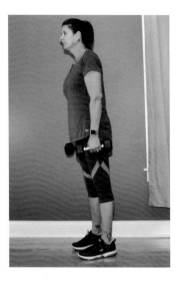 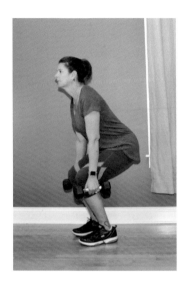

WIDE SQUATS

Stand with the feet wide, toes out at a slight angle and hold weights in front of the chest with the palms facing in. Keeping the knees in line with the toes, lower into a squat, keeping the knees back and abs in. Press into the heels, feeling it in your inner thighs and lower body to stand. Suggested weights: medium to heavy.

   1 x 12 reps

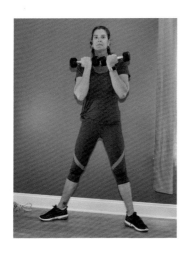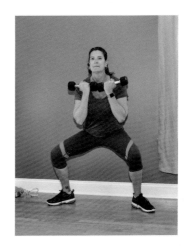

SIDE STEP SQUATS WITH BANDS

Loop the band around the feet and hold on to each handle. Take a wide step out to the right as far as you can, pulling the band up to create tension. Lower into a squat and then step back to start. Repeat, alternating sides.

   1 x 16 reps

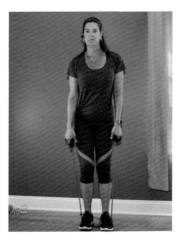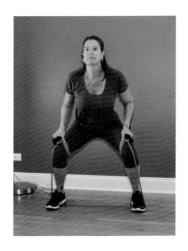

BAND REVERSE LUNGE

Loop the band under the right foot and curl the band up to create tension. Step back with the left foot into a lunge, taking the back knee straight down towards the floor. Step back and repeat for all reps before switching sides.

   1 x 12 reps

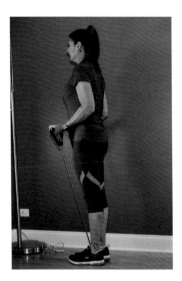 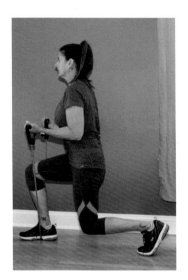

STATIC SIDE LUNGE

Hold a weight in both hands at chest level with the legs wide, toes facing the front of the room. Bend the right knee and send the hips back as you lower into a side lunge. Stand up and repeat, alternating sides. Suggested weight: heavy.

   1 x 16 reps

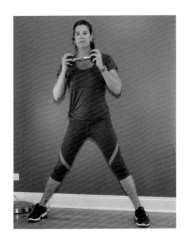 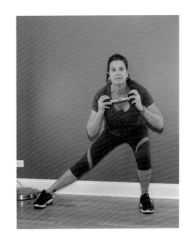

DEADLIFTS

Stand with the feet about hip-width apart and hold weights in front of the thighs. With the knees slightly bent, tip from the hips keeping the back straight and the abs in while taking the weight towards the floor. Keep the back flat and the weights close to the body like you're shaving your legs. Squeeze the butt to lift up and repeat. Suggested weights: heavy.

   1 x 12 reps

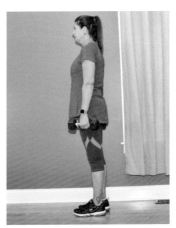 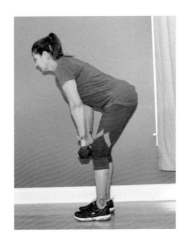

MARCHING BRIDGES

Lie face up on a mat with the knees bent and press the hips up into a bridge position. Holding this position, lift the right foot a few inches off the floor, knee bent. Lower the foot and repeat with the left foot, continuing to alternate sides.

1 x 16 reps

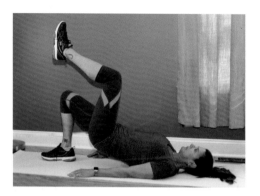 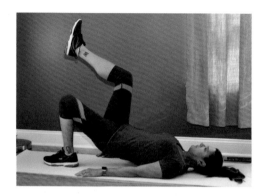

CRISSCROSS OUTER THIGH

While lying face up on the floor, loop the band around the feet and take the legs straight up in the air. Crisscross the bands, grab on to the handles, and pull the weight, resting the arms on the floor and keeping tension on the band. Open the legs out to the sides as wide as you can go, feeling it in the outer thighs. Return to start and repeat.

1 x 12 reps

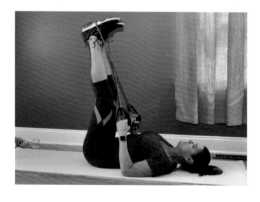 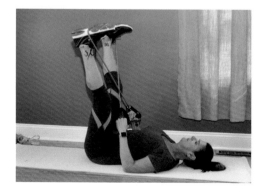

DEADBUG

Lie on the floor and lift the legs straight up in the air, pressing the feet together. While continuing to press the inside of your shoes together, bend the knees, taking them out to the sides as you bring the feet in towards your body, feeling it in the inner thighs. Keep squeezing the feet together as you press the legs back up and repeat.

1 x 12 reps

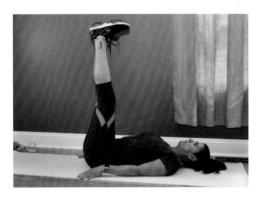 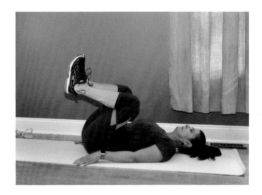

CHAIR HIP LIFTS

Lying face up on the floor, rest your lower legs on a chair. Flex the feet and press into the heels to lift the hips up, squeezing the glutes. Lower and repeat.

1 x 12 reps

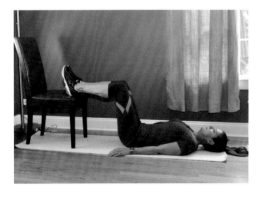 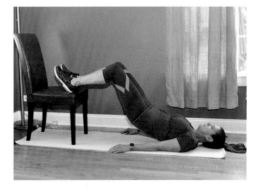

Chapter 12

Split Strength Training 2: Weeks 9 and 10

For the next two weeks, you'll take it to the next level with new upper and lower body exercises as well as a new core and balance workout. As with the previous workouts, begin with a warm-up and then do each move for the suggested reps and sets. Do one set during Week 9, and two sets during Week 10 skipping any exercise that causes pain.

EQUIPMENT NEEDED
Light, medium, and heavy weights
Light to medium tension resistance band
A sturdy, unmoving chair
A mat

SUGGESTED WORKOUT SCHEDULE
Day 1: Upper Body Strength 2/Flexibility
Day 2: Rest or active movement
Day 3: Lower Body Strength 2/Flexibility
Day 4: Rest or active movement
Day 5: Rest or active movement
Day 6: Core and Balance Workout 3
Day 7: Flexibility

UPPER BODY WORKOUT 2

ALTERNATING OVERHEAD PRESS
Stand holding weights in each hand with the arms bent, elbows at ear level, and arms like a goal post. Bracing the core, press the right hand up. Lower back to shoulder

level and then press the left hand up. Continue, alternating sides. Suggested weights: light to medium.

1 x 16 reps

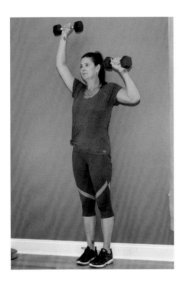 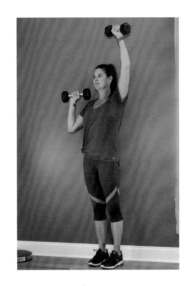

UPRIGHT ROWS

Stand holding weights in each hand, resting in front of the thighs with the palms facing the thighs. Bend the elbows and pull the weights up, taking the elbows just to shoulder level with the weights at chest level. Lower and repeat. Suggested weights: light to medium.

1 x 12 reps

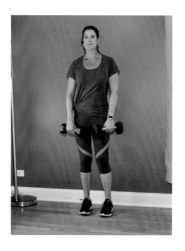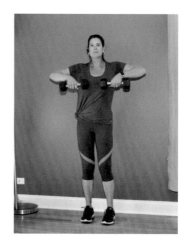

ONE WEIGHT FRONT RAISE

Hold a weight in both hands and take the right leg back in a staggered stance. Lift the weight straight up to shoulder level. Lower and repeat for six reps before switching legs. Suggested weight: heavy.

   1 x 12 reps

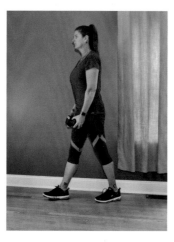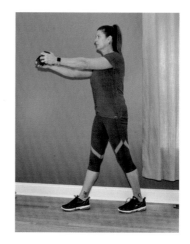

CROSS-BODY BAND BICEPS

Loop the band under the right foot and hold on to each handle. Use the left hand to keep tension on the band while you curl the weight up across the body with your right hand. At the top of the movement the palm should face the opposite wall. Lower and repeat for all reps before switching sides.

1 x 12 reps

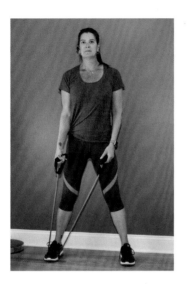 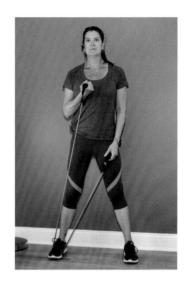

WIDE BICEPS CURLS

Hold weights in each hand with the shoulders rotated out, palms facing out. Keeping the hands wide, curl the weights up to the shoulders. Lower and repeat. Suggested weights: medium to heavy.

1 x 12 reps

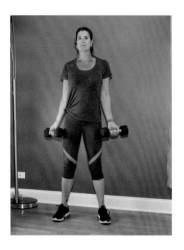 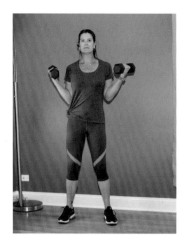

BAND HIGH ROWS

Loop the band under both feet and hold on to each handle with the palms facing back. Bend the elbows and pull the handles up so that your elbows are at 90-degree angles and parallel to the floor. This is targeting your upper back. Lower and repeat, adjusting where your hands are on the band to add or release more tension.

   1 x 12 reps

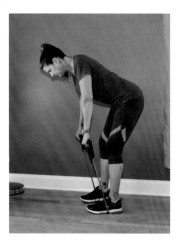 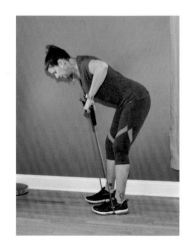

CHEST PRESS

Lie on a mat with the knees bent and hold weights straight up over the chest with the palms facing in. Keeping a slight bend in the elbows, open the arms out to the sides, gently lowering the arms until they just touch the mat. Return to start and repeat. Suggested weights: medium to heavy.

1 x 12 reps

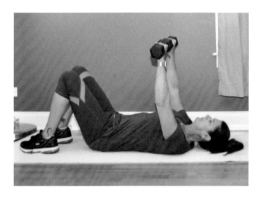 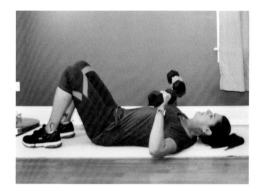

LYING TRICEPS EXTENSIONS

Lie on a mat face up holding weights in both hands straight up, palms facing in. Bend the elbows and bring the weights down to either side of the head. Squeeze the back of the arms and extend the arms straight up. Lower and repeat. Suggested weights: light to medium.

1 x 12 reps

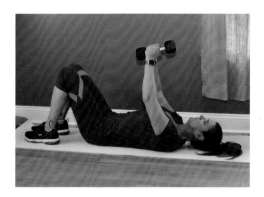 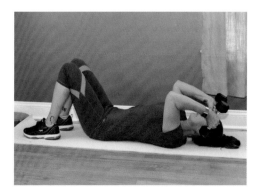

PULLOVERS

Hold one weight in each hand while lying face up on a mat. Keeping the elbows slightly bent, gently lower the weight behind your head, keeping your back flat on the floor. Lightly touch the weight to the floor and then squeeze the back to lift back up. Suggested weights: medium

1 x 12 reps

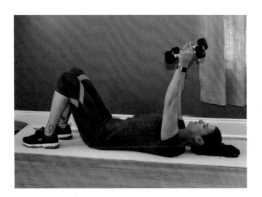 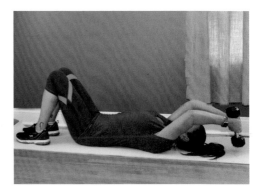

LOWER BODY WORKOUT 2

BAND SQUAT WITH SIDE LEG LIFT

Loop the band under both feet and hold the bands to create tension. Lower into a squat and, as you stand, lift the right leg up in a side leg lift. Lower the leg, repeat the squat, and do the exercise on the other side.

1 x 16 reps

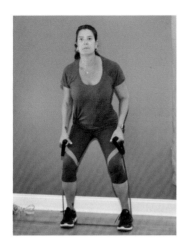 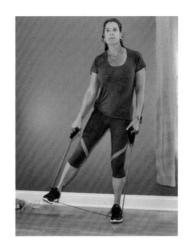

FRONT & BACK LUNGES

Hold weights in each hand with the feet together. Step forward with the right foot into a lunge, taking the back knee straight down towards the floor. In one move, step back with the right leg, taking it back into a reverse lunge.. Repeat for all reps, moving forward and back, before switching sides. Suggested weight: medium to heavy.

   1 x 12 reps

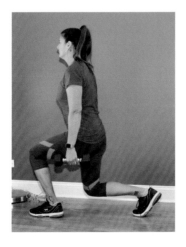 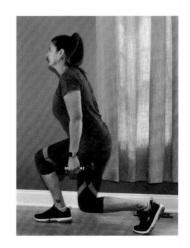

ONE-LEG DEADLIFTS

Standing, hold one weight in both hands and take the left leg back in a staggered stance. Keeping a slight bend in the front knee, tip forward from the hips, keeping the back flat and the abs in. Lower the weight towards the shoe, keeping the weight very close to the leg, until you feel a stretch in the back of the front leg. Return to start and repeat all reps before switching sides. Suggested weight: heavy.

  1 x 12 reps

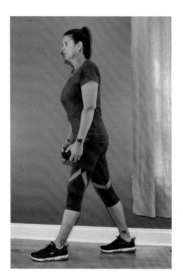 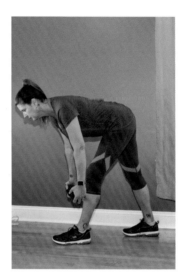

STEP OUT WIDE SQUATS

Stand with feet together and the weights at chest level, palms facing the chest. Step out into a wide squat with the toes out at an angle, going as low as you can. Step back and repeat the step out to the other side, continuing to alternate sides. Suggested weights: medium.

  1 x 16 reps

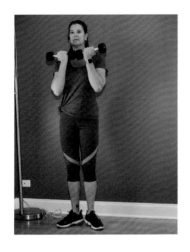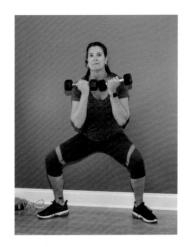

STEP OUT SIDE LUNGES

Hold a weight in both hands at chest level with the feet together. Step out to the right, sending the hips back into a side lunge, weight in the heel. Press back to start and repeat all reps before switching sides. Suggested weights: heavy.

   1 x 12 reps

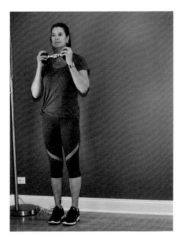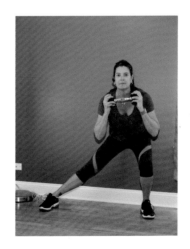

BAND LEG PRESS

Lying on the floor face up, loop a band around the right foot and grab on to the band close to your feet. Starting with the knee into the chest, press the right foot straight out towards the wall in front of you. Lower and repeat for all reps before switching sides. You may be able to use a heavier resistance band for this exercise.

   1 x 12 reps

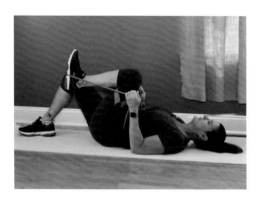 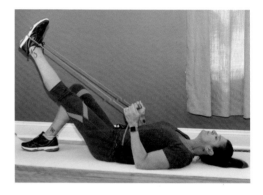

ONE LEG BRIDGE

Lying on the floor with knees bent, straighten the right leg straight up. Keeping the leg up, press into the left heel to lift the hips as high as you can. Lower and repeat for all reps before switching sides.

   1 x 12 reps

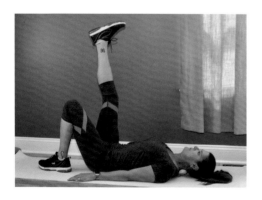 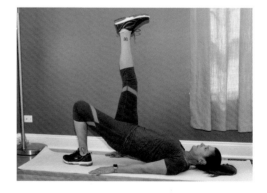

FLOOR LEG EXTENSIONS WITH BAND

Tie your resistance band around your ankles while seated, resting on the forearms with the abs in. Position the band over the top of the right foot and extend the leg, squeezing the front of the thigh. Lower and repeat for all reps before switching sides.

   1 x 12 reps

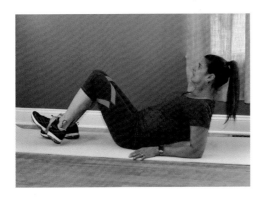 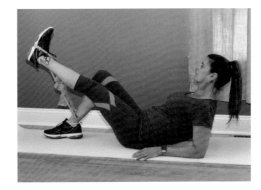

BUTT BLASTER WITH BAND

On your hands and knees, loop the band around the arch of the right foot, anchoring the handles on the floor with your hands. Starting with the knee into the chest, press the flexed right foot straight back. Lower and repeat for all reps before switching sides.

   1 x 12 reps

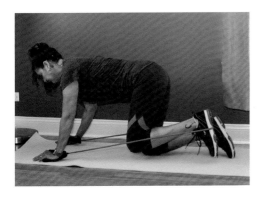 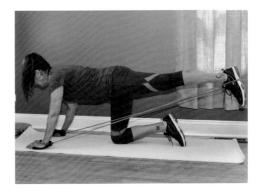

ONE LEG SLIDE

Start on the hands and knees and then straighten the right leg, placing the toe on a sliding device. Pressing the toe into the sliding device, slide the leg out to the side. Continue pressing down as you slide back to start. Repeat for all reps before switching sides.

1 x 12 reps

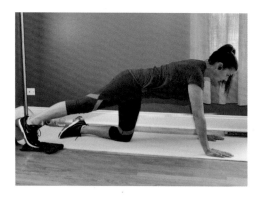 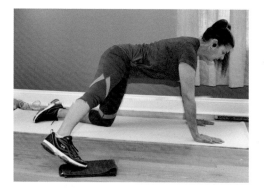

CORE AND BALANCE WORKOUT 3

CRESCENT KNEES
Begin standing with hands on the hips or on a chair if you need extra balance. Lift the right knee and then rotate the knee towards the right, then back down as though you're doing a half circle. Repeat for all reps before switching sides.

   1 x 12 reps

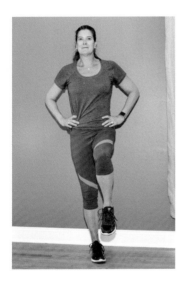 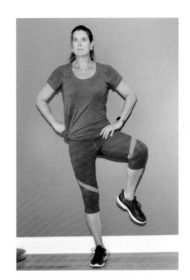

OPPOSITE ARM AND LEG LIFT
From a standing position, simultaneously raise the right arm up as you lift the left leg straight out to the side. Lower and repeat, alternating sides.

   1 x 16 reps

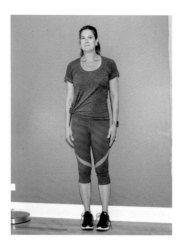 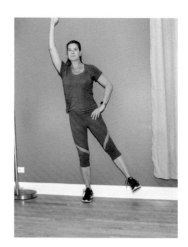

3-POINT TOE TOUCH

Hold on to a wall or chair for balance if needed and slowly take the right foot forward, touching the toe to the floor. Now bring the toe out to the side to touch the floor and then back behind you. Try to keep the leg up the entire time. Repeat for all reps before switching sides.

   1 x 12 reps

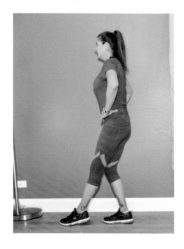 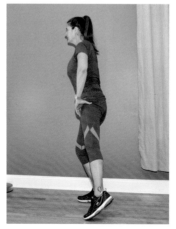 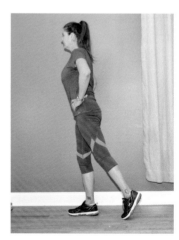

SINGLE STANCE SQUAT AND REACH

Stand with the weight on the right leg, resting on the tip of the toes. Bend the right knee and lower into a squat while lifting the left knee and reaching down with the left arm. Hold onto a wall for balance if you need to. Lift up and repeat for all reps before switching sides.

1 x 12 reps

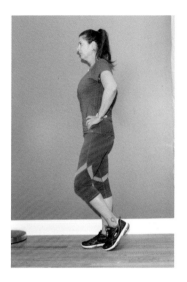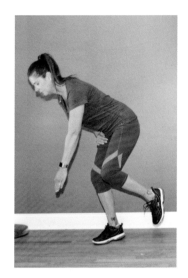

WALKING KNEE HUGS

Begin at one end of the room and take a step forward with the right foot. Bring the left knee up and hug it into the chest. Lower the left leg, step forward, and hug the right knee to the chest. Continue back and forth, alternating knees for three laps.

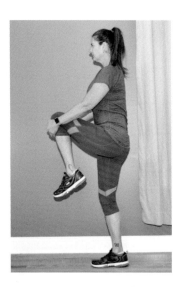
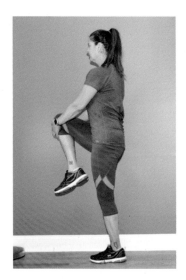

WALK OUT PLANKS

Begin on the hands and knees and slowly walk the hands out until your back is in a straight line from the shoulders to the knees. Slowly walk back and repeat.

   1 x 12 reps

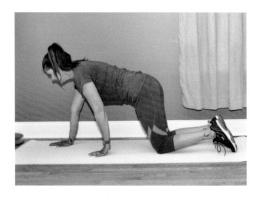
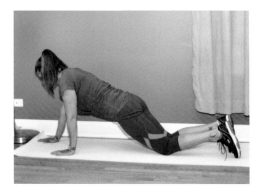

SIDE HIP LIFTS

Lie on your right hip resting on the forearm, knees and hips stacked. Keeping the knees on the floor, squeeze the abs to lift the hips off the floor. You can take the upper hand to the floor for support if you need to. Repeat for all reps before switching sides.

1 x 12 reps

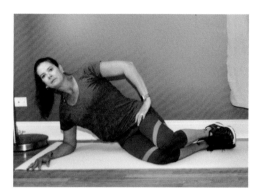 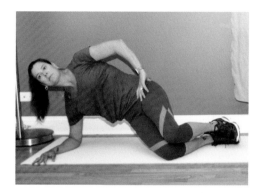

MODIFIED GET-UPS

Lie face up on the floor with the right knee bent, left leg straight, and the right arm straight up in the air. Press into the left forearm to push up, reaching the hand towards the ceiling. Lower and repeat for all reps before switching sides.

1 x 12 reps

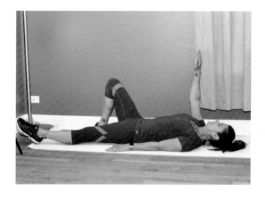 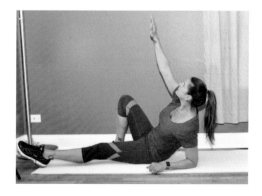

TOE TAPS

Lying on the floor face up with hands resting beside you, bring the knees up so that they're at about 90-degree angles. Contract the abs and slowly take the right foot towards the floor as low as you can. Lift and repeat, alternating sides.

   1 x 16 reps

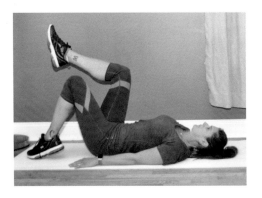 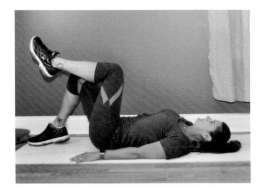

BACK EXTENSIONS

Lie on your stomach with the legs straight out behind you, arms bent and hands under the shoulders. Contract the abs and keep them tight as you lift the chest off the ground, gently using your hands if you need to. Lower and repeat.

   1 x 12 reps

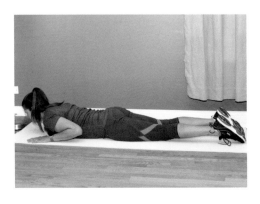 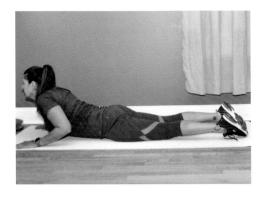

Chapter 13
Total Body Compound Strength Training: Weeks 11 and 12

Now that we've reached the end of the program, we're making more changes in order to challenge all the strength and balance you've accomplished. This workout takes everything you've learned and focuses on total body movements with an upper body and lower body component.

This is the ultimate way to train your body to be stronger and more functional in your daily life. As with the other workouts, make sure you warm up and do one set during Week 11, and two sets during Week 12, skipping any exercise that causes pain.

EQUIPMENT NEEDED
Light, medium, and heavy weights
Light to medium tension resistance band
A sturdy, unmoving chair
A mat

SUGGESTED WORKOUT SCHEDULE
Day 1: Total Body Compound Workout/Flexibility
Day 2: Rest or active movement
Day 3: Total Body Compound Workout/Flexibility
Day 4: Rest or active movement
Day 5: Rest or active movement
Day 6: Core and Balance Workout 3
Day 7: Flexibility

SIDE BAND SQUAT WITH BICEPS CURLS

Loop the band under the feet, holding handles in each hand. Step out to the right into a squat while curling the handles up to shoulder level in a biceps curl. Step back and repeat, alternating sides.

   1 x 16 reps

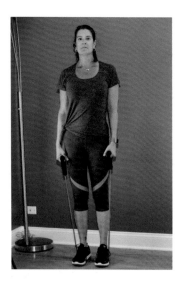
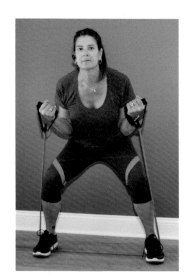

DEADLIFT WITH UPRIGHT ROW

Hold weights in front of the thighs and tip from the hips, back flat, lowering the weights towards the floor. Squeeze the glutes to stand and then pull the elbows up to shoulder level in an upright row. Lower the weights and repeat. Suggested weights: medium to heavy.

   1 x 12 reps

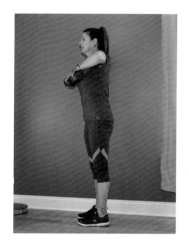 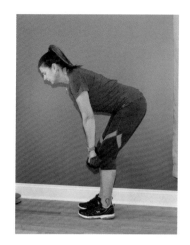

SQUATS WITH OVERHEAD PRESS

Begin standing holding weights just over the shoulders. Lower into a squat, sending the hips back while keeping the abs in. Press into the heels and, as you stand, press the weights overhead. Lower the weights and repeat. Suggested weights: medium.

1 x 12 reps

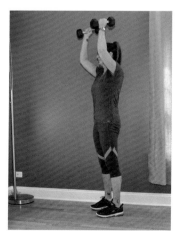 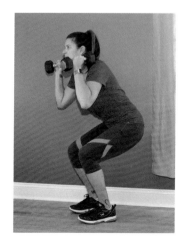

REVERSE LUNGE WITH LATERAL RAISES

Start with feet together and weights at your sides. Step back into a reverse with the right foot. At the same time, lift the arms out to the sides to shoulder level. Lower the weight as you step back in and repeat, alternating sides. Suggested weights: light.

   1 x 16 reps

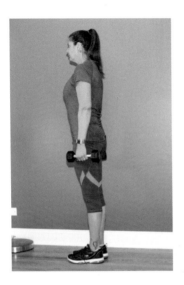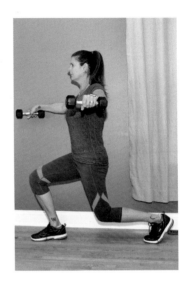

STEP BACK WITH ROWS

Start with feet together and weights at your sides. Step back with the right foot, bending the left leg and tipping from the hips with the back flat. As you step back, pull the elbows up into a double arm row. Lower the weights, step back, and repeat, alternating sides. Suggested weights: heavy.

   1 x 16 reps

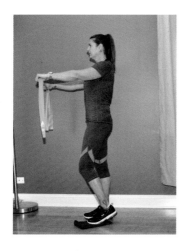
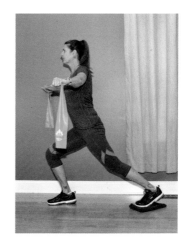

SLIDE REVERSE LUNGES WITH REAR BAND FLIES

Begin with the feet together, right foot on a sliding device and holding a resistance band straight out at chest level. Keep the weight in the left foot as you slide the right leg back. At the same time, open the arms out to the sides, squeezing the shoulder blades together. Return to start and repeat all reps before switching sides.

   1 x 12 reps

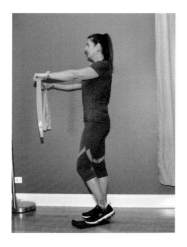
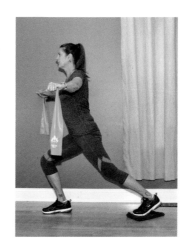

WOOD CHOPS

Hold a weight at chest level and step out to the right into a side lunge, sweeping the weight across your body and bringing towards the right wall. Step back while sweeping the weight diagonally up to the left. Repeat for all reps before switching sides. Suggested weight: light.

   1 x 12 reps

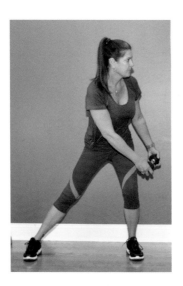 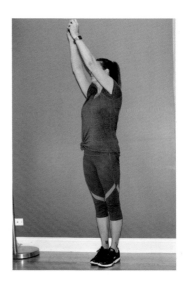

PUSH-UPS TO CHILD'S POSE

On the hands and knees with the back straight, lower into a push-up as low as you can. Press back as far as you can, stretching through the chest and back. Repeat, alternating a push-up and child's pose.

   1 x 12 reps

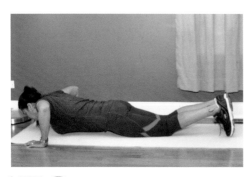 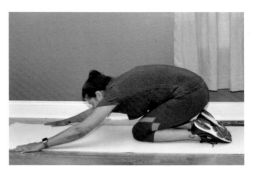

TRICEPS CORE KICKBACKS

On the hands and knees, hold a weight in the right hand. Pull the elbow up to torso level and contract the abs to keep your body stable. Straighten the right arm, taking the weight behind you and squeezing the back of the arm. Lower and repeat for all reps before switching sides. Suggested weight: medium.

1 x 12 reps

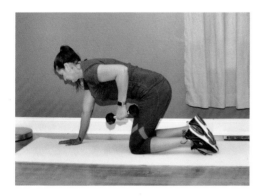 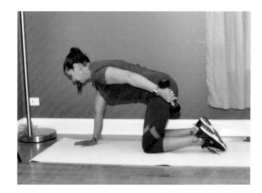

CHEST FLIES KNEES UP

Lie on the floor holding weights straight up over the chest, palms in. Take the knees up in the air, contracting the abs. Keeping the knees up, open the arms out to the sides, a slight bend in the elbows. Take the arms out to the side until the elbows touch the floor and then the arms back up over the chest. Suggested weights: light to medium.

1 x 12 reps

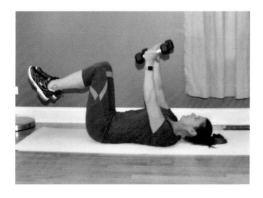 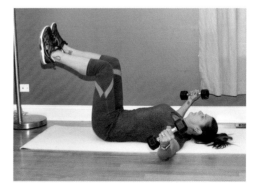

Chapter 14
What Happens Next?

However far you made it with the 12-week program, whether you got in every workout or not, the first thing you should do is to celebrate your success. Changing your daily habits and working your body are not easy things to do... if they were, everyone would do it, right?

Just some ideas include:

- ✓ A weekend getaway
- ✓ A night out
- ✓ A spa treatment like a massage
- ✓ Time reading your favorite book or listening to music
- ✓ Splurging on some new workout clothes

Celebrating is the way you mark what you've done as something worthwhile in your life. Something you've stuck with and something that made a difference.

Celebrating should be something that happens throughout the process, whether it's a small goal or a larger one.

But the real key to using exercise to your advantage involves two things: consistency and momentum.

You may hear people talk about staying motivated, but motivation usually isn't the first ingredient in the exercise mix. Being consistent with your workouts makes you more disciplined. Your body starts to expect that workout at 7:00 each morning and, as a result, it gets easier to do it.

That discipline adds to the next important ingredient which is momentum. Momentum builds as you increase that consistency and you get on a healthy lifestyle path that makes it easier to stick with.

So, what happens when you get to the end of this program? That doesn't mean you stop exercising! You have 12 weeks of practice that will help carry you into the future and maintain everything that you've gained over time.

First, it helps to get a broad view of the basic principles of strength training so you know exactly how to change your workouts when you're on your own.

MANIPULATING THE PRINCIPLES OF STRENGTH TRAINING

The underlying principles of strength training are what guide us in choosing every aspect of our workouts, from the exercises we do to the number of reps and sets we choose.

Once you have a broad view of these principles, you can use them to manipulate different elements of your workouts so you can keep making progress and keep things interesting, something you'll tackle on your own at this point.

THE OVERLOAD PRINCIPLE

You've learned that the only way to build strength and get better at something is to give your muscles more than they're used to handling.

This is important because the more your muscles do, the more they are capable of doing. That's why our bodies get sore when we change something; they have to adapt to those new challenges.

That means that, once you've built a basic foundation and mastered each exercise, as you did in this program, it's time to shift your focus to elevating your goals.

One important area here is concentrating on the amount of weight you're lifting. While the beginning of a strength training program is more about building a foundation, the next phase is about progressing and challenging yourself.

Focusing on your weights is where you'll take the next step, and you do that by this simple rule: Choose a weight that you can only lift for the desired number of reps.

In other words, you should be glad to get to that last rep and you should be able to do it with good form. But, that last rep should be challenging.

One rule of thumb is that, if you can keep going after the last rep of your set, increase your weight by about 5 percent. Since weights come in certain increments, you may not be able to do exactly 5 percent, which is just fine. Just increase the weight by what you have and adjust your reps so that you keep perfect form.

THE PROGRESSION PRINCIPLE

You've probably heard of plateaus, and that's one thing that happens when you don't change anything about your workouts. One thing you want to do is to continue to change things so that you're always progressing.

That's the underlying theme of this 12-week program as you conquer new and more challenging exercises as well as change the number of reps and sets you do over time.

SIMPLE WAYS TO PROGRESS

a. **Changing your reps**—The rep ranges for your 12-week program generally stay between 12 and 16 reps to give you an easy-to-follow strength training recipe. However, you can progress and change your workouts by a) adding more weight and reducing your reps to around 8 to 10 or b) reduce the weight you're using and increase reps to 16... beyond that number you won't see much of an improvement unless you're doing body weight exercises such as push-ups.

b. **Changing your sets**—In this program, you do 1 or 2 sets depending on the workout. You can take these workouts to another level by adding a set, taking it up to 3 sets per exercise, making sure you rest in between. When you change to a different workout, you may start with fewer sets and increase over time.

c. **Changing the type of resistance**—In this program, we use bands and dumbbells for a variety of exercises. You can also use things like medicine balls, gym machines, barbells, or any other type of resistance to change how an exercise feels and how your muscles work.

d. **Changing your exercises**—Another way to progress is to change the exercises you do, much like in this program. For example, during the first two weeks, you did wall push-ups. Eventually, you progressed to modified push-ups on the floor. You could progress that further by doing push-ups on your toes. Even the simplest change counts, such as standing on one leg while doing a biceps curl or even sitting during an exercise instead of standing.

THE REVERSIBILITY PRINCIPLE

This principle is the very reason for this chapter, because it's all about the fact that if you don't use it, you lose it. Research shows that just a month off from exercise can reverse all the good things you achieved, which is why you have to keep using those muscles.

Exercise isn't just a means to an end, but an ongoing journey, and you should consider it part of your daily lifestyle, just like brushing your teeth or taking a shower. And realize that sometimes, you can exercise on a regular basis and sometimes you can't.

It could be a physical issue or something that happens in your life but, chances are, it will happen. But you can always start again.

With that in mind, it's wise to have some ideas of how to keep that momentum going.

THE SPECIFICITY PRINCIPLE

This is probably one of the easier principles to keep in mind because it has to do with what you want to accomplish.

This principle, simply said, is that you do what serves you the best. For example, if I have a client who loves to garden, I focus more attention on those areas: Squatting, bending, pulling, and digging.

Another client might want to run a marathon, which involves an entirely different type of training.

The key is to think about what you want to get out of life every day and specifically the movements those tasks require and then focusing on strengthening those movements.

TIPS TO KEEP GOING

- ✓ Keep to a schedule—Keep planning your workouts on a regular basis so they're a part of your life, just like a doctor's appointment. Plan them out and put them in your calendar.
- ✓ Mix things up—You have weeks of workouts and exercises to choose from and, with your newfound strength, you may be ready to venture out and try other activities. Cross-training with other activities keeps your body and mind strong in new and different ways.
- ✓ Don't be afraid to experiment—While the program may seem regimented, once you get a basic foundation of strength you can push your limits a little. Try doing the workouts in reverse order or group exercises together. It's easy to get stuck in a rut sometimes, so make an effort to change things on a regular basis.
- ✓ Keep exploring—One great thing about the time we live in is that information is at our fingertips. You can often find free videos on the Internet, community group fitness classes, and other resources to tap into to make things more interesting.
- ✓ Remember what you've learned—Strength training is a learning experience as well as a time to connect with your body in a different way. Keep that connection with your body going.

Most importantly, consider exercise as your own personal Fountain of Youth that will keep you strong and independent. Focusing on your quality of life is a great way to stay motivated in taking care of your body, for the present and for the future. The great thing is that your body knows what you need. Listen to it.

References

American College of Sports Medicine. *ACSM's Guidelines for Exercise Testing and Prescription*. Philadelphia, PA: Wolters Kluwer, 2018.

Arnold, C.M., R.A. Faulkner, and N.C. Gyurcsik. "The Relationship between Falls Efficacy and Improvement in Fall Risk Factors Following an Exercise Plus Educational Intervention for Older Adults with Hip Osteoarthritis." *Physiotherapy Canada* 63, No. 4 (2011): 410–20. https://doi.org/10.3138/ptc.2010-29.

Bryant, Cedric X., Sabrena Newton-Merrill, and Daniel J. Green. *ACE Personal Trainer Manual*. San Diego, CA: American Council on Exercise, 2014.

Bryant, Cedric X., and Daniel J. Green. *ACE Personal Trainer Manual: the Ultimate Resource for Fitness Professionals*. San Diego, CA: American Council on Exercise, 2003.

Fragala, Maren S., Eduardo L. Cadore, Sandor Dorgo, Mikel Izquierdo, William J. Kraemer, Mark D. Peterson, and Eric D. Ryan. "Resistance Training for Older Adults." *Journal of Strength and Conditioning Research* 33, No. 8 (2019): 2019–52. https://doi.org/10.1519/jsc.0000000000003230.

Jankowski, C.M. "Resistance Exercise for Muscular Strength in Older Adults: A Meta-Analysis." *Yearbook of Sports Medicine* 2011 (2011): 407–10. https://doi.org/10.1016/j.yspm.2011.03.064.

Lavin, Gary. "Efficacy of Weight Training: Multiple Sets versus Single Sets." *Strength and Conditioning Journal* 21, No. 3 (1999): 17. https://doi.org/10.2165/00007256-199826020-00002.

Liu, Christine K., and Roger A. Fielding. "Exercise as an Intervention for Frailty." *Clinics in Geriatric Medicine* 27, No. 1 (2011): 101–10. https://doi.org/10.1016/j.cger.2010.08.001.

McGrath, Chris. "Core Training for Injury Prevention - ACE." American Council on Exercise, 2012. https://www.acefitness.org/education-and-resources/professional/expert-articles/2906/core-training-for-injury-prevention/.